The
Diabetic's
Book

Also by June Biermann and Barbara Toohey
The Woman's Holistic Headache Relief Book
The Diabetic's Sports & Exercise Book
The Diabetes Question & Answer Book
The Diabetic's Total Health Book

Under the name Margaret Bennet
Biking for Grownups
Cross-Country Skiing for the Fun of It
How to Ski Just a Little Bit
The Peripatetic Diabetic
Dr. Owl's Problem
From Baedeker to Worse
Alice in Womanland

Published by J. P. Tarcher, Inc.
LOS ANGELES

Distributed by Houghton Mifflin Company
BOSTON

The Diabetic's Book

ALL YOUR QUESTIONS ANSWERED

June Biermann and Barbara Toohey

Foreword by Diana Guthrie, R.N.
Diabetes Nurse Specialist

The authors would like to thank the following authors and publisher for
permission to reprint material:
For the recipe on pages 54–55, Copyright © 1979 by Rose Dosti, Deborah
Kidushim, and Mark Wolke. Reprinted by permission of Harper & Row,
Publishers, Inc.

Library of Congress Cataloging in Publication Data

Biermann, June.
    The diabetic's book.

    Bibliography: p. 245
    Includes index.
    1. Diabetes—Miscellanea. I. Toohey, Barbara.
II. Title.
RC660.B459   616.4′62   81–50792
ISBN 0–87477–197–8   AACR2

J. P. Tarcher, Inc.
9110 Sunset Blvd.
Los Angeles, Calif. 90069
Library of Congress Catalog Card No.: 81–50792

Design by Barbara Monahan

MANUFACTURED IN THE UNITED STATES OF AMERICA

S 10 9 8 7 6

First Edition

To Jackie Tippen, who over the last twenty years
has given us the two greatest gifts:
love and work.

CONTENTS

Short Subjects   113

FOR INSULIN-DEPENDENT DIABETICS   153

The Big Questions   154

Short Subjects   169

FOR CONCERNED FAMILY MEMBERS AND FRIENDS   177

The Big Questions   178

Short Subjects   190

FOREWORD

AS A DIABETES NURSE SPECIALIST, I HAVE FOUND very few books to recommend without reservation to those who need information on diabetes. This is the one book I would unhesitatingly recommend above all and to all. It has something for everyone: for the person with diabetes—whether on diet alone, diet with pills, or especially diet with insulin— and for family members and friends who want to help.

There is another group of people I would encourage to read this book: the health professionals—those of us who guide, support, and direct the persons with diabetes and their family members. Often, we as professionals look at those with whom we come in contact from the textbook side. It is too seldom that we can take the time to explore the feelings and thoughts of family members or the one living with diabetes. This book gives us an important glimpse of the "other side." In fact, student nurses as well as other health professional students should read this book as a required part of their preparation, not only for what it shares about diabetes but also for its awareness of the thoughts and emotions of any person having a chronic illness.

17

The Diabetic's Book is filled with fact and fancy, with pathos and humor. In its informal yet scientific approach it covers material not touched on in most patient education manuals. It does not overemphasize the problems that can be associated with having diabetes but it does put them in a knowledgeable perspective.

June has shared many of her experiences in previous books, as well as in the first edition of this question-and-answer book. One of the key messages in the book for the person with diabetes is, "Well, if June did it, so can I." And of particular interest for concerned family members and friends is the section in which Barbara shares her experiences in living for one month as if she had diabetes and suggests that family members of a person with diabetes try this same thing themselves.

The message of these questions and answers, overall, is hope: hope through research, hope through planning, and hope through the best self-care possible. The questions asked are down-to-earth, everyday questions, those you might ask of a health professional or of someone else who has diabetes. The answers express various sides of the questions, as is appropriate, and include anecdotes both informative and humorous.

I especially like the reflection that refers to the need of health professionals to practice what we preach. In fact, it has made me feel guilty enough about my sometimes too many "off," rather than "on," health care practices. I intend to turn over a new leaf in life, especially if I can keep a copy of this book at my bedside.

I am reminded of my favorite lecture given by Barbara Toohey and June Biermann. They discuss one of the most important medical prescriptions: "four hugs a day." This book represents one of the hugs: the ability of these two people to share themselves with others. The other three hugs, to be dispensed after reading this book, involve sharing your newfound understanding, communicating your hope—and completing

the prescription by getting as well as giving these hugs daily
for the rest of your life.

Diana Guthrie, R.N., M.S.P.H., F.A.A.N., C.
Diabetes Nurse Specialist
University of Kansas School of Medicine—Wichita

ACKNOWLEDGMENTS

WE OWE OUR THANKS TO THE FOLLOWING PEO-
ple who helped us find the answer to the question of how to
get this book written:

Andrea Almasy, the Bio-Dynamics sportswoman who practices what we preach;

Mary Ellen Baran, the world's only exdiabetic and an in-
spiration to us all;

Richard K. Bernstein, who'll soon have the medical creden-
tials to match his innovative and exhaustive knowledge of
diabetes;

Ron Brown, diabetes counselor and product expediter at the
Sugarfree Center, who gave us released time to write;

Marion Craig and her Magic Typewriter, who performed repeated manuscript emergency rescue operations;

Lucinda Dyer and Mary Lou Brady, who keep the fruit of our
labor from dying on the vine;

Janice Gallagher, who puns us into action and flails more
out of us than we think is there;

Diana Guthrie, our living question-and-answer book—we
sleep better nights knowing that she has checked out our
manuscript;

Theresa Miller, who relived her problems as a brittle diabetic so that others might not have to repeat them;

21

Kathy Noone, the Ames representative whose highest priority is helping diabetics;

Lee Schulman, our English connection, who dealt us a Glucometer in the nick of time;

Esther Shuster, the Pittsburgh Diabetes Educator who educated us on the G. T. Injector;

The Valley College Library Staff, who put up with our absences—and our presence;

Diane Victor, the Valley Presbyterian diabetes nurse educator whose down-to-earth approach leads diabetics to upbeat lives;

Helen Way, when there's no Way, there's no way we can get time off for R & R after meeting deadlines.

All things are difficult
before they are easy.

—THOMAS FULLER, 1608–1661
Gnomologia No. 560

INTRODUCTION

THE JUNE HALF OF OUR WRITING TEAM WAS diagnosed diabetic fourteen years ago. Although it was not the worst of times to become diabetic, it was not the best of times either. Practical help for those with this health problem was scarce. The now active and growing American Association of Diabetes Educators did not even exist. The available books were ponderous and discouraging.

Because of this lack of help and information, we started devoting the largest portion of our time to finding strategies for coping with diabetes. Using June as a guinea pig, we constantly checked out new angles of attack on the problems of diabetes. In exchanges after our talks before diabetes associations and in correspondence with hundreds of other diabetics and health professionals, we have continuously learned more. We shared our newfound information in our previous books on diabetes: *The Peripatetic Diabetic* in 1969, *The Diabetes Question & Answer Book* in 1974, *The Diabetes Sports & Exercise Book* in 1977, and *The Diabetic's Total Health Book* in 1980.

And now here is *The Diabetic's Book*. We felt there was a
need for this, our fifth book on the subject, because there has
never been a period in the history of diabetes in which so
many new discoveries have been made and so much new information has become available. We know that the majority of
diabetics are not aware of these breakthroughs that can make
their lives easier, happier, healthier, and *longer*.

Another motivation for this book came from the Sugarfree Center for Diabetics. This is a mail-order service we
started two years ago to supply learning materials and new and
hard-to-find diabetes care products at minimum cost and max-
imum convenience. The Sugarfree Center has put us in contact
with over 5,000 diabetics and their families and with many
doctors, nurses, and dietitians specializing in diabetes. All of
these people have shared with us their insights, inspirations,
and innovations in handling diabetes. We want to bring all this
new knowledge to you.

Finally, our earlier basic book, *The Diabetes Question & Answer Book*, is now both out-of-date and out-of-print. Many diabetics and diabetes educators have encouraged us to write a
replacement. In researching, writing, and living this book, we
have kept in mind that, to replace our *The Diabetes Question &
Answer Book*, it must be able to serve as a teaching text for use
in educational programs. In writing style and organization,
therefore, we have been guided by the expressed needs of diabetes nurse educators and teaching dietitians and social workers. We have aimed for readability and accuracy plus a touch of
fun and a feel for the human condition. We hope that the book
will prove to be a flexible learning tool equally useful with
groups and individuals and that the diabetes teaching teams
will find *The Diabetic's Book* compatible with their unique creative classroom techniques.

To provide direct and quick access to information we have
divided the book into three sections: (1) questions and answers
for everyone, (2) questions and answers for insulin-dependent

diabetics, and (3) questions and answers for family members and friends.

We have further divided each of these sections into two parts: The Big Questions and Short Subjects. The Big Questions are conversational exchanges in which we amplify and clarify the information that everyone needs to know. In the Short Subjects we provide answers to the many and varied personal questions that individuals have asked us over the years. For further ease of approach there is a detailed index.

In the Reference Section at the back of the book, you will find a Directory of Services for Diabetics, Exchange System Meal Plans, Brand Name Exchanges, How Sweet It Is, Injection Sites, Insulin Onset, Peak and Effective Duration chart, Glucagon Injection (for emergency treatment of insulin shock), Insulin Reaction Information, and Suggested Reading.

All in all, we feel that if you have to become diabetic this is the best time in the history of the world for it to happen to you. Never before has it been so totally possible to learn how to keep your blood sugar normal, to avoid and/or minimize the once-feared complications of diabetes, and to enjoy life as it was meant to be enjoyed. With this book we want you to learn how to live better with diabetes and *through* diabetes.

SOMETHING
FOR
EVERYONE

ALTHOUGH THIS SECTION OF THE BOOK IS IN-tended for everyone involved with diabetes—both newly diagnosed and experienced diabetics, whether insulin, pill, or diet controlled; family members; friends; and health professionals—it is aimed primarily at beginners.

Why for beginners? For two reasons. The first reason was born one day when June was emerging from her dentist's office. The door to a neighboring internist's office opened and a man came out. He was clutching a copy of the American Diabetes Association's approved diet. He had obviously just been given The News, because in 96-point headlines his face was printed with the negative emotions of confusion, fear, and despair. June could read them easily because they were the same emotions she'd seen in the mirror on her own D (for diagnosis) day. While writing this section of the book, we've kept this man's face before us. Our goal has been to change his expression—and that of all newly diagnosed diabetics—to one of understanding, courage, and hope.

The second reason for aiming this section at beginners is based on the Zen theory of the expert's mind versus the beginner's mind. Since the expert's mind thinks it knows everything, the expert's mind is closed to new ideas. It knows what can't be done. It thinks in terms of limitations.

The beginner's mind, on the other hand, is still open. To the beginner all things are possible. Not even the sky is the limit.

We hope that the following information will help all of you—no matter how many years you've had diabetes or worked in the field of diabetes—to become beginners again.

≡ THE BIG QUESTIONS ≡

How can I keep from being depressed over my diabetes? _____

It's not easy. It's only logical to be depressed when you first learn you have diabetes. And all the cheerful remarks people make about how much nicer it is to have diabetes than leprosy or than being run over by a moving van or some such nonsense do no good at all. You know that it's *not* better than having nothing wrong with you.

After all, you have to make many, many changes in your life, and at first glance, these changes all seem to be for the bad. On top of that, you feel like an outcast. You're no longer like everyone else. Of course, no one ever *is* like everyone else, but at the moment you feel like the town pariah, and you're certain that all your friends are going to drop you now that you have diabetes.

You get the automatic "why me?" reaction. "Why should *I* be selected to get this rotten disease?" "Why should *I* be threatened with blindness or kidney failure or gangrene or an early death if I don't follow a rigid regime?" Why indeed? There's really no reason. It's just the breaks of the genetic game. As a doctor told us once at a meeting, "Every person carries around about forty-four genetic defects." One of yours happens to be diabetes, and the fact is that some people draw out far worse tickets than diabetes in the genetic lottery. But that doesn't make you feel any better. As A. E. Housman said, "Little is the luck I've had and, oh, 'tis comfort small, to think that many another lad has had no luck at all."

So what do you do about all this? You can sit and resentfully mutter about cruel fate and wallow in your woe, or you can, as the old saying has it, take the lemon you were handed and make lemonade out of it. We read an article about a woman who is a successful author and consumer advocate on radio and TV in Los Angeles. She described her beginnings: "When we married, during the early years it was rough. We were poor, but I wasn't about to go on welfare. So I decided if I wanted clothes, I had to make them. If I wanted the best bread I'd better learn how to bake. What I did was take poverty and turn it into an art."

What you need to do is take diabetes and turn it into an art. Do all the things you need to do for your diabetes and make them enhancements to your life.

How do I turn diabetes into an art?

The beginning step is to accept the fact that you have diabetes. The first thing most people do with diabetes is to deny it. Oh, your mind may know you have diabetes, but everything else about you—your heart, innards, soul, imagination, all those things you really listen to—say, "This has nothing to do with me. I'll ignore it and it will go away."

Alas, it won't, and you'll never be able to practice the art of diabetes until you get rid of the idea you don't have it. As a matter of fact, you need to do more than just accept your diabetes. One young woman, after hearing us speak at a diabetes meeting, said to June, "You actually seem to embrace diabetes." That she does. Not that she wouldn't prefer not to have diabetes, but since she does have it, she's determined to squeeze all the good out of it she can.

What's good about having diabetes?

Without being ridiculously Pollyannaish about it, we can affirm that diabetes *does* do some positive things for you. This isn't just our idea. Many diabetics have written to us and told us about what they consider to be the advantages of diabetes.

For one thing, you learn the principles of good health. Until you're whammed with something dramatic like diabetes, you may just bumble along wrecking your health through bad habits, laziness, and ignorance. Diabetes teaches you the right way to live and gives you a reason for doing so. As one diabetic skier put it, "This disease, this condition will keep you healthy and fit for whatever your heart desires. I feel I'm better off because I'm not fat; never have I been out of shape, and I eat well and thoughtfully."

Diabetics often actually feel better than they did before having their disease. Young diabetics have reported to us that they do better in sports than their nondiabetic friends because they never eat junk food and always keep regular hours. They're in top-notch shape all the time. They also say they're less susceptible to the colds and flus that their friends pick up with seasonal regularity.

Diabetics often look better than their nondiabetic contemporaries. Conscientious diabetics are lean and vital and bright of eye and quick of step. People of the same age who don't have diabetes to goad them onto the path of healthful living often are pudgy, sallow, and lethargic.

Diabetes develops your self-discipline. Young persons who have diabetes and must assume responsibility for their own care develop a mature attitude of self-sufficiency at an early age. The discipline of following the diabetic way of life carries over to school and work and sports and creative endeavors. It can help make you a successful person in all areas of living.

Sometimes diabetes even sparks ambition. We know a young diabetic woman who is a successful city attorney. She told us how her choice of a profession came about.

"When I got diabetes in high school I knew I'd have it all the rest of my life. I realized it would be an expensive disease and I decided I wanted to always be able to take care of myself—and take care of myself *well*—whether I ever got married or not. That's why I worked hard to prepare myself for a good career."

And having diabetes makes you more compassionate toward others with problems. You learn how to give help gracefully and receive help without embarrassment or resentment. This, after all, is what puts the humanity in human beings.

But perhaps best of all, diabetes makes you capable of change. To change is the hardest thing for people to do. That's why so many of us take the easy way out and stick in a rut for our entire lives, unable to rouse ourselves into action to make the changes that could make us into the persons we were meant to be.

Diabetes, because it requires changes, and rather dramatic changes at that, shows you that you *can* change. If you can change in one area, then you are capable of change in other areas. You can improve not only your health but your whole life.

But so much of the change seems to be giving up pleasures. How can I feel good about that?

We found that when June, in her early fits of depression, was ticking off all the pleasures she'd have to give up because of diabetes, what she was really ticking off were habits. Something like eating a sweet dessert was a habit that she considered a pleasure merely because she'd done it so often that it was a comforting part of her daily routine. The trick is to establish new *good* habits and turn them by constant use into pleasures.

This is not as hard as you may think. Eating a delectable, juicy piece of fresh fruit can become as much of a habit-pleasure as eating a big, gloppy dessert. For many people a daily bike ride or after-dinner walk is a pleasurable habit, and it can become one for you, too.

Furthermore, when you're thinking of the things you have to give up because of diabetes, think of these: you have to give up ever waking up with a hangover, either of the cigarette or alcohol variety; you have to give up discovering on a shopping trip that you've ballooned another dress or suit size; and you have to give up feeling like a sluggish blob because of lack of exercise.

Finally, if, as you make the changes in your life, you still have moments of depression, try to keep in mind that it's part of the human condition to be depressed from time to time. There will be a natural tendency for you to lay your every woe on the doorstep of your diabetes. That's unfair to diabetes. Bad though it may be, it's not enough of a villain to be responsible for every dismal moment in your life. Even if you didn't have diabetes, you wouldn't be frisking around in a constant state of ecstasy. Though they call life the human comedy, it isn't all laughs for anybody.

How do I start making all the changes I have to for my diabetes?

Again, that's not a question with easy answers. Every time we go to a meeting of diabetes educators, the major topic is "Compliance." We don't really like this word because it sounds as if you should bend to the will of the doctor or nurse or dietitian who knows what's good for you, and you, you misbehaving rascal, refuse to comply. Actually, nobody can make you "comply," can force you to change your habits. That has to come from within. The late psychologist Abraham Maslow has explained that you can only reach the point of change after you pass through several emotional stages in a "hierarchy of needs."

First, you have to have your basic physiological needs met. That is, you must have food to eat and a place to stay. We'll presume you have that. Then you have to feel safe. This one's often a problem when you're first diagnosed because, far from feeling safe, you feel threatened. When you've conquered that fear, you need to have feelings of belonging and love from others. Many times the love and belonging are there, but newly diagnosed diabetics don't realize it. They think that friends and family members will reject them because of their "flaw." After you recognize how wrong you were there, then you need to develop or redevelop your feelings of self-esteem and self-love, realizing you're a good person who is worth taking care of, worth going to the trouble of *changing* for the better. Only when you reach that point can you make those difficult changes.

Let's take you back to step two, the place where you feel threatened, unsafe, and afraid. Most, if not all, of your fear is fear of the unknown. Although people may have been throwing a lot of miscellaneous diabetes information at you, you

probably haven't caught a tenth of it. Let's go back to the diabetes basics. As you learn them—really learn them this time—
your fears should gradually dissolve. Without fear clouding
your vision, we think you'll be able to see you haven't been
abandoned and you'll become ready to accept the love that's all
around you. You'll begin liking yourself—diabetes and all—
again and, lo, you may find the needed changes in your life
almost start making themselves.

What is diabetes? _____

Diabetes is a physical problem that causes you to have too
much sugar in your blood. The medical name for it is *diabetes
mellitus.* The first word, *diabetes,* is from Greek and means "to
run through a siphon." The second word, *mellitus,* is from
Latin, and means "honey." The two words together are usually
translated "sweet water siphon." (In case you don't speak Greek
and Latin, *diabetes mellitus* is pronounced *dye-uh-**beet**-ease
mell-**eye**-tus.*) The doctors in ancient times called it that because
they noticed that diabetics urinated a great deal and their urine
tasted sweet. Yes, *tasted* sweet. In those days the only way a
doctor could test urine was by tasting it. (And doctors today
won't even make house calls!)

What makes the urine sweet?

When blood sugar goes too far above normal, some of the
sugar spills over into the urine so the body can get rid of it.
(That's why you sometimes hear diabetics say, "I'm spilling
sugar," or just, "I'm spilling.") The point at which this happens
is called the *renal threshold.* Normally sugar spills between blood
sugar levels of 150–180, but it can vary from person to person
and even from time to time in the same person. And the older
you get the higher your renal threshold goes. You may not

spill sugar into your urine until your blood sugar is well over 200. (For example, June starts spilling at about 220.) The opposite is true of children. They often have lower-than-normal renal thresholds.

Why is there too much sugar in the blood?

The cells of the body run on a fuel called *glucose*. This is the sugar that the body manufactures from the food we eat. Glucose is carried to the cells in the bloodstream. But the body cells are locked up tighter than a Manhattan apartment. Glucose can't get into a cell without a key. That key is *insulin*. Insulin is a hormone that comes from a gland called the *pancreas*.

In the case of diabetics who must take insulin, the pancreas is either no longer making any insulin or not making enough of it. That is to say, all or some of the keys (insulin) may be missing. On the other hand, in those who don't require insulin often there are plenty of keys or even too many, but the cells either do not have enough locks (called *insulin receptors*) to let the insulin in, or something is keeping the locks from working. For example, they may be gummed up with fat.

What's wrong with having high blood sugar?

High blood sugar is an indication that your body is getting little or no fuel. In desperation it begins to convert its own fat and muscle into fuel. This is like chopping down the walls of your house to get wood to burn in your fireplace. If you keep that up, soon you have no house left.

But that's not even the worst of it. When the body burns itself for fuel, excess *ketones* (substances which are formed during the digestion of fat) are given off. These excess ketones can poison the body. This poisoning—called *ketoacidosis*—can lead to death.

Perhaps you remember reading about the California boy Wesley Parker, whose father threw away his insulin because a faith healer had "cured" the boy's diabetes. Within three days Wesley was dead from ketoacidosis.

There is still something else wrong with having high blood sugar. Let's say you have *some* insulin that's working—either insulin you've injected or insulin you've produced in your own pancreas—but you don't have enough. Then, while you won't use up your own body as fuel and you won't be poisoning yourself with ketones, you still have too much glucose flowing through your bloodstream. That's not good, because this situation brings about long-range diabetes complications like blindness, kidney failure, and gangrene of the feet.

Do we have to talk about complications?

We have mixed emotions about ranting at you about diabetes complications. Some doctors and nurses feel that unless they paint vivid horror pictures, diabetics won't take their disease seriously and do what they should to take care of it.

Sometimes this backfires, though, as we learned in a letter from one diabetic. On the first day of her diagnosis and hospitalization, she was told by the head nurse, "You have a dreadful, dreadful, dreadful disease." The nurse convinced her that all she had to look forward to was "becoming a blind, bilateral amputee, carried off to dialysis three times a week." This experience so affected her psychologically that

> I lay awake night after night shaken with an unbearable fear. It permeated every aspect of my daily life. I gave up

wearing contact lenses because I cried so much. I was worn out emotionally. My college doctor suggested psychiatric counseling. I was hesitant, but after six months was helped greatly and I started taking better care of myself because I finally felt there was a glimmer of hope for the future.

On the other hand, you can't just ignore or gloss over complications. They can happen, but as the latest studies are revealing, you *can* avoid these complications, if you keep your diabetes in control—that is to say, you keep blood sugar normal most of the time.

What's normal blood sugar? _____

The normal range is around 60 to 120 (milligrams of sugar per deciliter of blood), depending on the method used to test the blood sugar. The objective of all diabetes treatment is to keep blood sugar within this range. After you eat, blood sugar rises and reaches its peak between one-half and one hour later. Even in nondiabetics the blood sugar varies according to times of eating and what is eaten. Rarely, however, does it go over 150. Blood sugars above 160 suggest the person is diabetic.

Here is the normal pattern of blood sugar for nondiabetics in relationship to meals:

RELATION TO FOOD	BLOOD SUGAR RANGE
Fasting (before breakfast)	60–100
1 hour after meal	100–140
2 hours after meal	80–120
3 hours after meal	60–100

At the Kansas Regional Diabetes Center in Wichita, good control of blood sugar is measured by the following standard:

RELATION TO FOOD	BLOOD SUGAR
Fasting (before breakfast)	105 ($\pm$10%)
1 hour after meal	140 ($\pm$10%)
2 hours after meal	120 ($\pm$10%)
3 hours after meal	110 ($\pm$10%)

These figures are for capillary blood tests. Some physicians' reports are based on blood plasma, which gives readings 10 to 15 percent higher than whole blood. If you take your own blood sugar at home with chemically treated strips (see Something for Everyone: How Can I Tell If My Diabetes Is in Control?) and a prick of the finger, you'll be using capillary blood.

Can anything besides eating and not eating make my blood sugar go up or down?

Blood sugar often goes up when you have an infection—the flu, the common cold, stomach upsets. Major surgery and pregnancy cause a rise. Then there are a number of drugs that tend to raise blood sugar. Caffeine, oral contraceptives, estrogen, and cortisone are the most important to know about. Emotional tension also causes blood sugar to swing upward.

Besides being lowered by fasting or by insufficient food, blood sugar goes down when you exercise strenuously. Among drugs with a lowering effect are alcohol (when you don't eat while drinking), large doses of aspirin, blood-thinning drugs, barbiturates, and sulfonamides.

Is it all right to have low blood sugar?

No. Low blood sugar can be very hazardous for a diabetic because you become irritable, befuddled, uncoordinated, and, in extreme cases, unconscious.

Usually only insulin-taking diabetics experience low blood sugar, although non-insulin takers who are losing weight sometimes have periods of low blood sugar or, as it's also called, *hypoglycemia*.

Isn't hypoglycemia a separate disease?

It's both a condition and a disease. As a disease, hypoglycemia is almost the opposite of diabetes. The pancreas produces too much insulin, which causes the blood sugar to plummet. Strangely enough, hypoglycemia can be a precursor of diabetes.

What caused me to get diabetes? ___

Researchers have been puzzling over the answer to this question for decades. They have more leads now than ever before but still not many definite answers. We'll summarize points of what is known and you'll have to try to apply them to yourself.

First, diabetes runs in families; so whether you got it as a child (only 4 to 5 percent of all diabetics do) or later in life, you still had to have some genes that predisposed you to it. Second, some physical or emotional stresses combined with your hereditary tendency and pushed you over the brink into diabetes.

If you got diabetes as a child (the commonest age to be diagnosed is around twelve), recent studies show that a virus related to the mumps virus might have brought on your diabetes by damaging your pancreatic cells that produce insulin (*beta cells*). Or maybe something went wrong with your immune system and your body itself destroyed some of these cells.

For those diagnosed in mid-life or later, the number one diabetes-triggering stress is excess weight. Some 80 to 85 percent of those diagnosed are overweight. Another influence is aging and a general slowing of body functions. In fact, more cases of diabetes are diagnosed after the age of sixty than at any other time of life. Of all people over sixty-five an astounding 30 percent have diabetes or impaired glucose tolerance (they cannot maintain normal blood sugar levels).

Overproduction of certain hormones—growth hormone from the pituitary, thyroid hormone, epinephrine, cortisone, and glucagon—makes the body's insulin less effective and can also bring on diabetes.

Pregnancy, which makes additional demands on the body, can cause diabetes to develop. In fact, some women show diabetes symptoms during pregnancy but their symptoms disappear after the baby is delivered. Mary Tyler Moore wasn't that lucky. Her diabetes was diagnosed shortly after a miscarriage and from then on she has been insulin-dependent.

Surgery or a major illness can activate diabetes. June became diabetic not long after a hysterectomy.

And finally, emotional stress can be implicated. It can be either long-term, grinding stress such as chronic unhappiness with a job or a family situation, or it can be a sudden extreme emotional shock. The well-known author of diabetic cookbooks, Jeanne Jones, became diabetic almost immediately after her husband was killed in an automobile accident.

I always thought you could get diabetes from eating too many sweets. Isn't that true?

No. A lot of people have that mistaken idea. Diabetes is sometimes even called "sugar diabetes," which adds to the confusion. Diabetes can't be caused by eating too much sugar, except when your diabetes was triggered by overweight and you became overweight from eating too many sweets. But even in that case, it wasn't specifically the sugar that was to blame. Diabetes could have developed if you ate too much of anything and gained weight.

Will I have to take insulin? _____

That depends to a large extent on the kind of diabetes you have. Lately it's been recognized that diabetes is really more of a family of diseases than just one disease. If you get diabetes as a child or young person (this used to be called *juvenile diabetes*) you almost certainly will have to take insulin, because your pancreas is making little or no insulin. If, however, you get diabetes later in life—say, after forty—you're usually overweight, and often if you get your weight down you can be virtually symptom-free without insulin.

What if you're not overweight but you get diabetes after forty? Do you have to go on insulin or not?

You may or you may not. You're a fence straddler. June was one of these. She was diagnosed at the age of forty-five. She was not at all overweight (5'5" and 116 lb.) and never had been. Her doctor put her on pills at first (Tolinase). They worked for her for several months. Then, although she followed her diet meticulously, she began running high blood sugar again. What's worse, her weight dropped to 108 and she started producing those calling cards of totally-out-of-control diabetes, ketones. To get her blood sugar down, she had to start taking insulin and has been taking it ever since.

The French divide their diabetics not into age groups but rather into the thins and the fats. They believe that if you're thin when you're diagnosed you'll probably have to take insulin and if you're fat, you won't. This certainly has held true for June.

If you once start taking insulin, do you have to take it for the rest of your life?

If you're a juvenile diabetic, yes, you're probably stuck (!) with it. Occasionally after children or young people are first diagnosed and start using insulin, there comes a honeymoon period. The disease seems to fade away, they can stop taking insulin, and their family believes a miracle has occurred and they are cured. Not so. Like all honeymoons, the diabetes honeymoon eventually comes to an end and insulin injections must begin again. (But enjoy it while it lasts.)

Sometimes if you're an adult-onset diabetic you may be on insulin only until you get your weight down.

Also, diabetics who aren't normally on insulin may have to take it when they're sick or have an infection or are pregnant. Then when they're well again, or the baby is delivered, they can stop.

Finally, Dr. James Anderson at the University of Kentucky has discovered that with his HCF diet (see Something for Everyone: What Is the Diabetic Diet?), many adult-onset diabetics taking fewer than twenty units of insulin a day are able to stop taking it altogether. Juvenile diabetics can expect to lower their insulin dosage by about one-fourth on the HCF diet.

Can you take insulin in pill form?

Insulin is not available as a pill. It is a protein, and the stomach would digest it the way it digests a lamb chop. Insulin must be measured into a syringe and injected by needle. That's how every insulin-dependent diabetic does it, except for the few who own a needleless injector that jet sprays it in (see For Insulin-Dependent Diabetics: How Can I Get Over My Fear of the Needle?).

The future may hold better news. Scientists are working to perfect an encapsulated insulin pill that can pass through the stomach without being digested. And, hear this: At the Hebrew University in Jerusalem, they have had success with insulin in suppositories. The question we have with this innovation is: would it really be all that much more convenient to, for example, insert an insulin suppository before dinner at a restaurant?

What are the pills that some doctors prescribe for diabetics? _____

The pills that some adult diabetics take have the trade names Orinase, Tolinase, Diabenese and Dymelor. They are called *oral hypoglycemics*. Oral means you take them by mouth; hypo means low, and glycemic refers to blood sugar. Put that all together and you have a pill that lowers blood sugar.

These pills work by making the person's own pancreas produce more insulin. Only diabetics who are still making some insulin on their own can use them. If you are the type of diabetic who can't keep your blood sugar normal on diet and exercise alone, your doctor may consider you a good candidate for these drugs. However, many doctors and diabetics prefer to go directly to insulin rather than experimenting with the drugs first. There are several reasons why.

No one knows if the drugs are safe. Since the 1970 study by the University Group Diabetes Program, many physicians have stopped prescribing the oral hypoglycemics, because this research revealed that they may increase the risk of dying from heart disease. The FDA has even issued a statement on the dangers of side effects of the pills. This must be distributed with them.

The pills have also been accused of causing weight gain, the very thing an adult diabetic generally doesn't need.

Another problem is that certain diabetics have a temporary success with the pills, as June did, and then the pills stop working for them. In that case, there is nothing to do but switch to insulin. (One great advantage of insulin is that over the last sixty years it has proven itself to be perfectly safe.)

How can I decide whether or not to take the pills?

The decision is up to you and your doctor. We agree with those physicians who prefer insulin to pills, unless, of course, the diabetic is blind or has some other problem that would make injecting insulin difficult. And we urge you, if your doctor wants you to take the pills, not only to participate fully in the final decision, but to make a special effort to control your blood sugar by diet and exercise alone. (Have you really lost all the weight you should and are you really eating the best diet?)

If you do opt for the drugs, be sure to get explicit information about how the particular one you take interacts with other drugs you may be taking. Oral hypoglycemics do not mix well with alcohol, as they prevent alcohol from being broken down by the body, and you may experience flushing, nausea, rapid heartbeat. Other drugs that interact with the pills are

steroids (trade name: Prednisone), estrogens, fluid pills, pheny-
toin (Dilantin), propanolol (Inderal), and decongestants. For
complete information check your drugs out with your phar-
macist or in the book *The People's Pharmacy* by Joe Graedon (see
Suggested Reading).

Above all, don't make the mistake of using the pills as a
substitute for willpower. June once watched in horror as another diabetic slurped his way through a hot fudge sundae.
When she shrieked at him, he winked, popped a pill into his
mouth, and said, "That'll take care of it."

A final word of caution. Don't rely on a drug and urine
tests for diabetes control. Have frequent blood sugars taken either at home or in your doctor's office. Or have a regular
every-three-months *glycohemoglobin* (see Something for Everyone: How Can I Tell If My Diabetes Is in Control?). Many
people on pills coast along with high blood sugar for years
without even knowing it because of their high renal threshold.
This is what has come to light in our dealings with older diabetics at the Sugarfree Center.

Can my diabetes be cured? _____

Things are looking up. Scientists are working on a number of
promising possibilities.

1. A mechanical pancreas. What they're aiming for is
one about three inches in diameter, approximately the size of a
heart pacemaker, that can be implanted. That's a pretty small
package to contain all the good things they need to put in it: a
glucose sensor to report the blood sugar level, a laboratory to
analyze the findings, a computer to calculate how much insulin is needed, a reservoir of insulin that can be released in the
proper quantity into the bloodstream, a pump, a fail-safe device
to counteract the release of too much insulin, and a power supply for the whole operation.

By way of a progress report, we can tell you that Dr. J. Stuart Soeldner of the Joslin Research Laboratory is perfecting an implantable sensor that reads blood sugar levels and sends a signal to a transmitter to activate an insulin pump. At present the sensor has been reduced to the size of a nickel.

2. Beta cell transplants. The beta cells are the part of the *islets of Langerhans* in the pancreas that produce insulin. During the first experiments with animals, these cells were implanted in different parts of their bodies with only short-term success. Lately, researchers under Dr. Paul Lacey in St. Louis have had longer-lived success by injecting rat cells into the large vein that leads into the liver in diabetic mice. The insulin-producing cells are first cultured for seven days below body temperature to prevent the immune reaction from being triggered.

3. Immunization. Juvenile Diabetes, like polio, may someday be virtually eliminated with immunization shots that prevent the virus from attacking the insulin-producing cells of the pancreas.

4. Genetic change. This is science fiction stuff, but it may be the ultimate solution to diabetes along with every other human genetic flaw. It is a theory that some day when all the mysteries of genetic structure are solved, some sort of genetic surgery to correct genetic defects will be found.

5. Pancreas transplants. There are with these, as with heart transplants, the two problems of getting the necessary organ and keeping the body from rejecting it after it's transplanted. Even so, over 100 transplants have been made in the United States and some have not been rejected. One young South Carolinian, thirty-five-year-old Mary Ellen Baran, has had a double transplant: pancreas and kidney. She had been diabetic for twenty-three years when in 1972 she had a successful kidney transplant and then in 1978 a successful pancreas transplant at the University of Minnesota hospital. She is now cured of diabetes.

We had breakfast with Mary Ellen in Atlanta and watched in amazement as she relished her pancakes and syrup. She confessed that "within three months of leaving the hospital, I had tasted every dessert known to man and gained fifteen pounds." She now has a grip on her new freedom and her weight is back to normal. "My meal plans are *exactly* as they were before the operation," she told us. And believe it or not, she says she eats less refined sugar now than she did as a diabetic!

Keep watching the papers. You'll be seeing a lot of headlines like "Diabetes Cure in Sight." Unfortunately, when you read on, you'll probably discover that the "fantastic" breakthrough has been with three mice in New Jersey.

In time, however, we're confident the real cure will come. What you have to do in the meantime is keep your spirits up, keep your diabetes in control, and keep yourself in the best possible shape so that you'll be able to, as Mary Ellen puts it, "hop onto your own star when it comes your way."

Will diabetes shorten my life? ____

In the past the statistics about the shortened life expectancy of diabetics have been, to say the least, depressing. But now there's more upbeat news. For instance, since 1970 the death rate for diabetes has *declined* about 21 percent. The decline appears to be due to a decrease in cardiovascular deaths among diabetics. (About 60 to 70 percent of diabetics die of cardiovascular disease.)

The old estimate of life expectancy for diabetics was that, all things being equal, diabetes shortens a person's life by one-third. Frankly, not only is this figure now outmoded by the above statistics, but we consider it far too drastic for an in-control diabetic. But just for the sake of argument, let's accept it. What, then, does "all things being equal" mean?

Our interpretation is that if you do *not* have diabetes and yet you live the way diabetics do—you eat a perfectly balanced diet low in fats and sugar; you drink little or no alcohol; you do not smoke; you keep your weight slightly below normal; you get regular daily exercise and regular nightly sleep—then you will live one-third longer than a diabetic doing the same thing.

But let's face it. Without the incentive of a chronic health problem to make them follow such an optimum lifestyle, 99 people out of 100 won't do it. No, better make that 999,999 out of 1,000,000.

Now, let's say all things *aren't* equal. You don't have diabetes. You are overeating—and eating all the wrong things—overdrinking, oversmoking, and carousing around and never exercising, except possibly in occasional violent weekend spurts. Will all this shorten your life? Yes, very likely more than diabetes will.

We can't offer any guarantees, but as Dr. Oscar Crofford of Vanderbilt University pointed out at the 1980 ADA annual meeting, we already know that poorest control of diabetes is associated with highest risk of complications, while near-perfect control is associated with the lowest risk. So if you follow the recommended diabetic lifestyle, keep your blood sugar in good control and your risks down, it is our unshakable belief that you can bring your span of years up to and even beyond that of the average person who is either unaware of the principles of good health or disinterested in following them. Like the Lord, diabetes giveth as well as taketh away.

A concrete testimonial to our theory is that over 500 people have been awarded the Fifty Year Duration of Diabetes medal by the Joslin Diabetes Foundation in Boston. The medal is given to people who have successfully lived fifty years or longer as insulin-dependent diabetics. This is a considerable achievement, because many people who earn the medal got diabetes before insulin was available. This means their early years with diabetes were particularly dangerous and detrimental. These people are the true heroes and heroines of diabetes. And there would be many, many more medal winners except that the Joslin Foundation has such stringent requirements of complete medical records.

There is also a Quarter Century Victory Medal given for twenty-five years of living with diabetes. It is awarded only to those who are "in superb condition," that is to say, totally free of complications (normal eyes, kidneys, blood pressure; no hardening of the arteries). Approximately 200 persons have received this medal.

Naturally, if you ignore your diabetes and the good health principles it requires you to follow, you can make all the depressing statistics come true. So the real question is, "Will *I* shorten my life?" And only you can answer that one by the way you follow the diabetic program of diet and exercise.

What is the diabetic diet? _____

You hear a lot of talk about "the diabetic diet" and we ourselves sometimes fall into the trap of using that term. In reality, though, there is no one diabetic diet.

In the first place, it's not a diet in the way most people think of one—a rigid and unnatural eating pattern that you follow until you remove extra pounds, at which time you revert to your old way of eating and almost invariably put the pounds back on again.

If it's not a diet, then what is it?

It's more of a calorie-controlled meal plan to guide you into good lifetime eating habits. And happily it's a meal plan with almost infinite variations to suit your lifestyle, taste, and ethnic heritage.

You may have heard of the Exchange Lists for diabetics. These are food lists created by the American Diabetes Association and the American Dietetic Association specifically to help diabetics control the number of calories they eat and plan balanced meals. They divide all foods into six groups: (1) Milk, (2) Vegetables, (3) Fruit, (4) Bread and Starchy Vegetables, (5) Meat, and (6) Fat. At each meal you are allowed an assigned number of choices (called "exchanges") from most of the groups.

For example, if you're allowed a choice from the Bread and Starchy Vegetables list, you can select one slice of bread or one-half bagel or one tortilla or one-half cup of rice or one small potato or one-third cup corn or one-half cup winter squash or any other "exchange" on that list. (There are a total of seventy-four foods to choose from on this one list!)

Let us give you some examples of a total meal. Say you're supposed to eat 1,800 calories a day. These are what exchanges you might be allowed for dinner:

3 meat exchanges

3 bread exchanges

2 vegetable exchanges

1 fruit exchange

2 fat exchanges

1/2 nonfat milk exchange

Here are some of the possibilities on that plan for meals:

Meal Example No. 1

Chicken, baked	3 oz.
Peas	½ cup
Rice	½ cup
Roll, yeast, plain	1
Tomatoes	1 cup

Applesauce	½ cup
Margarine	1 tsp.
Italian dressing (for tomatoes)	1 tbsp.
Skim milk	½ cup

Meal Example No. 2

Halibut, broiled	3 oz.
Lima beans (1 exchange—1/2 cup)	1 cup
Biscuit, 2-inch diameter	1
Asparagus	1 cup
Strawberries	1 cup
Tartar sauce	2 tsp.
Margarine	1 tsp.
Skim milk yogurt (to top strawberries)	1/2 cup

Meal Example No. 3

Lasagna* (3 meat, ½ bread, 1 vegetable, 2 fat)	2-inch × 3-inch piece
Bread sticks	6
Popcorn	3 cups
Lettuce, pepper, mushroom salad	free
Cantaloupe, 6-inch diameter	¼ melon
Skim milk yogurt with herbs (nonfat dressing for salad)	½ cup

*Recipe follows. From *Light Style,* by Rose Dosti, Deborah Kidushim and Mark Wolke (San Francisco: Harper & Row, 1979), p. 127.

Lasagna Recipe

This lasagna goes light on fats and starch to help lower the calories.

8 ounces lasagna noodles
1 pound ricotta cheese (made from partially
    skimmed milk)
6 tablespoons egg substitute, or 2 eggs
⅛ teaspoon ground nutmeg
2 tablespoons minced parsley
3 cups Italian Meat Sauce
1 pound mozzarella cheese, shredded
½ cup grated Parmesan cheese (optional)

Cook lasagna until just tender. Drain, rinse, and let stand in cold water. Beat ricotta cheese with egg substitute or eggs. Stir in nutmeg and parsley. Cover the bottom of a 9-by-13-inch, nonstick baking pan with a 1/4-inch layer of Italian Meat Sauce. Top with a layer of half the noodles and add half of the remaining meat sauce. Spread half of the ricotta cheese mixture over meat sauce and sprinkle with half of the mozzarella cheese. Repeat layers, ending with mozzarella cheese. Sprinkle evenly with Parmesan cheese if desired, and bake at 375 degrees F. for thirty-five minutes, or until cheese melts and is golden.

Makes sixteen servings.

Each 2-by-3-inch piece with Parmesan cheese contains about:

257 calories
264 mg sodium
12 g fat
53 mg cholesterol (content unavailable for lasagna
    noodles)
Exchanges: 1 vegetable, 3 meat, 1/2 bread

Italian Meat Sauce

Use Italian plum tomatoes when in season for best flavor and texture.

2 pounds ground beef sirloin
2 large onions, chopped
3 cloves garlic, minced
10 Italian plum tomatoes, peeled and diced, or 1 (20-ounce) can low-sodium tomatoes, diced
1 (16-ounce) can low-sodium tomato juice
1 tablespoon dried oregano, or 3 tablespoons chopped fresh oregano
1 teaspoon dried thyme, or 1 tablespoon chopped fresh thyme
1/2 teaspoon dried marjoram, or 1 1/2 teaspoons chopped fresh marjoram
2 teaspoons fennel seeds
1 teaspoon dried basil, or 1 tablespoon chopped fresh basil
1 bay leaf
3/4 cup chopped parsley
1/2 teaspoon pepper
1/2 cup dry red wine (preferably Chianti)

Combine meat, onions, and half the garlic in a large saucepan. Sauté until onions are tender and meat is crumbly. Add tomatoes, tomato juice, remaining garlic, oregano, thyme, marjoram, fennel, basil, bay leaf, parsley, and pepper. Bring to a boil, reduce heat, partially cover, and simmer two hours, stirring occasionally. Add wine and simmer thirty minutes longer, stirring occasionally. Remove bay leaf.

Makes about 6½ cups.

NOTE: It is necessary to peel the tomatoes to make a thick sauce.

Each 1/4-cup serving contains about:

81 calories

24 mg sodium

1 g fat

30 mg cholesterol

Exchanges: 1 meat, 1/2 B vegetable

You can see what immense variety you can have using the Exchange Lists. If your doctor hasn't given you a copy of the Lists, you can order them from the American Diabetes Association for fifty cents (see Reference Section: Directory of Services for Diabetics). They can also be found in *The Diabetic's Total Health Book* (see Suggested Reading). Then the best thing for you to do is have a dietitian take the chart in the Exchange List booklet, fill in the total number of exchanges on your individual eating plan, and indicate how they should be divided into meals and snacks. (For examples of how this is done, see Reference Section: Exchange System Meal Plans.)

I didn't notice anything but fruit for dessert on these meals. Aren't there any dessert exchanges?

No, there aren't. What you have in place of dessert is fruit or maybe occasionally a small serving of ice cream or a very small piece of very unsweet cake. In other words, you can't have concentrated sweets and that's what most desserts are.

What do you mean by concentrated sweets?

Concentrated sweets are what, when you taste them, are sweet, all sweet, and nothing but sweet. They're sugar, honey, and syrup. They're candy, frosted cake, pies, cookies, and ice cream sundaes. They're almost everything listed on restaurant menus as desserts. They're all soft drinks, except artificially sweetened ones.

Concentrated sweets are an assault upon your system that sends your blood sugar soaring. Besides that, they quickly use up your daily allotment of calories without giving you any real food value in return—empty calories, they're known as.

How do I know how many calories a day I should be eating?

As with so many other things with diabetes, you'll have to experiment to a certain degree. Your doctor will probably tell you the number of calories he or she thinks you need in order to lose or gain weight or stay the same as you are. Your doctor can't know, however, how active you are and how efficiently your body burns food and will have to raise or lower the calories if your weight doesn't go in the direction it needs to.

Table 1 (page 58) can be used as a general guideline.

Do all diabetics follow the Exchange Lists?

No, there are other possibilities. Dr. James Anderson of the University of Kentucky has developed the HCF diet. HCF stands for high carbohydrate/high fiber. This diet is also extremely low in fat. It is inexpensive, healthy, and good for weight reduction. It also helps to lower and stabilize blood sugar. The Exchange Lists for this diet are available in *User's Guide to HCF Diets*. (Order from HCF Diabetes Foundation, 1872 Blairmore Road, Lexington, Kentucky 40502, or from the Sugarfree Center.)

Some unstable juvenile diabetics working toward tighter control use a low carbohydrate/high protein and fat diet in conjunction with daily blood sugar testing and multiple shots of insulin. We *know* this diet is the opposite of the HCF diet,

TABLE 1
CALORIE ALLOWANCE FOR ADULTS FOR VARIOUS BODY WEIGHTS AND AGES, ASSUMING LIGHT PHYSICAL ACTIVITY*

Median Body Weight of Men		Daily Calorie Allowances According to Age			Median Body Weight of Women		Daily Calorie Allowances According to Age		
lb	kg	22	45	65	lb	kg	22	45	65
110	50	2200	2000	1850	88	40	1550	1450	1300
121	55	2350	2150	1950	99	45	1700	1550	1450
132	60	2500	2300	2100	110	50	1800	1650	1500
143	65	2650	2400	2200	121	55	1950	1800	1650
154	70	2800	2600	2400	128	58	2000	1850	1700
165	75	2950	2700	2500	132	60	2050	1900	1700
176	80	3050	2800	2600	143	65	2200	2000	1850
187	85	3200	2950	2700	154	70	2300	2100	1950
198	90	3350	3100	2800					
209	95	3500	3200	2900					
220	100	3700	3400	3100					

*Data from Food and Nutrition Board, National Academy of Sciences, National Research Council: Recommended dietary allowances, ed. 8, Washington, D.C., 1974, U.S. Government Printing Office, p. 29.

but different diets work best for different diabetics. Vive la différence! This beats the old days when all diabetics were treated the same. Now you and your dietitian can choose the diet plan that suits both your needs and your taste.

What are these carbohydrates and proteins and fats?

They are the basic food elements. Bread, cereal, vegetables, and fruit are mainly carbohydrates. Poultry, fish, meat, cheese, and eggs are mainly protein. Butter and cooking oil are fats. Many foods are combinations of all three food elements. Whole milk, for example, has carbohydrate, protein, and fat, and so do peanuts.

Does everyone feel as confused as I do about what I can eat?

Naturally. Deciding what to eat is for most people the most confusing part of adjusting to diabetes. You really need some special help at first. A dietitian can help you most. A dietitian will know all the dietary possibilities available to you and will be able to write out meal plans to get you started. When you have questions—as you inevitably will—you'll have the dietitian to turn to. In the beginning of your diabetes days (daze?), your dietitian will be as important to you as your doctor.

How can I find a dietitian?

If there isn't one on your doctor's staff, ask for a recommendation or call the local hospital and ask them for a recommendation.

You might also get in touch with the local affiliate or chapter of the American Diabetes Association. If they can't help you, write the American Dietetic Association or Consulting Nutritionists for a list of names of dietitians in your area (see Reference Section: Directory of Services for Diabetics).

Sometimes dietitians are listed in the yellow pages of the telephone directory. They may be listed under the term nutritionists as well. But you have to be careful. There are some strange types who call themselves nutritionists and they may try to put you on seaweed and soybeans and promise you the moon (that is to say, a cure). Stay away from these at all costs and their costs are likely to be high—the moon is an expensive commodity.

Make sure the dietitian is an R.D.—a registered dietitian. And try to find one who has enough imagination and knowledge to open up meal possibilities geared to your own tastes and needs and not one who just gives the same food prescription to all diabetics.

Will I be able to follow my diet in restaurants?

Of course. It won't be as easy as following it at home where you can select and measure everything to make sure you're getting exactly what you need, but with a little experience and ingenuity it can be done. In fact, it is done by diabetics every day.

At first, when you're just getting started with diabetes, you might want to check out the restaurant ahead of time to see what they have on the menu that would be right for you. This gives you time in advance to figure out what you want to order. You can also find out if they have, for example, fruit for dessert rather than something gloppy and sweet. If they don't you can bring along a piece of fruit and either eat it there or eat it after you leave

Checking out the restaurant ahead of time is also a good idea because you'll know if it's open or not. Sometimes on a trip June has gone out to a restaurant recommended in a travel book or article only to find it's been closed for six months. This can be more than an awkward situation if it's time to eat and there's no other restaurant around.

For insulin-dependent diabetics, a reservation is very important. The person taking the reservation should be informed that one of the diners is a diabetic and that the table *must* be ready at the time of the reservation and the food *must* be served without undue delay. (None of this sitting around in the bar for an hour waiting for the table the way a lot of restaurants do to try to get you to buy a bunch of extra drinks!)

What kinds of things should I order in restaurants?

As long as you avoid concentrated sweets, you can usually order anything you want. At first, though, try to avoid unfamiliar concoctions that are likely to have a lot of sauce (sauces often contain a great deal of carbohydrates and fat). Straightforward meat, poultry, or fish, and potatoes and vegetables are the easiest things to recognize and measure.

This doesn't mean that you're forever stuck with plain fare. As you gain more experience, you'll be able to do more daring dining in ethnic restaurants. Actually, it won't be daring at all if you do a little cookbook research on the various ethnic dishes. When you know what's in a dish—say *pasta e fagiole* or *blanquette de veau* or beef in oyster sauce—you'll know whether or not it's a good idea for you. In time you'll also learn to eye-measure your food and know how much of a certain dish you can eat.

What do I do if they serve too much food?

Leave what you can't eat or, in the case of expensive protein, take it home with you in a doggie bag. (You may have enough meat to last you for two or three meals!)

You should also watch for the restaurants that have special "light eater" dinners. There aren't many of these, but there are more and more all the time, because more and more people want to watch their weight or, as in the case of older people, just have diminished appetites. Another possibility for getting smaller portions is to ask if you can have the children's dinner. Restaurants are sometimes willing to serve it to adults if you pay a small surcharge. It will still be less than paying for the gross regular portions.

Our favorite trick for getting smaller portions and saving money and yet experiencing the best of dining out is to go for lunch rather than dinner. The portions are about half as large with prices to match. A further advantage is that you're eating your main meal in the middle of the day so you can walk it off afterward rather than just going to bed on a full stomach and letting it turn to fat. We do this main-meal-at-lunch trick when we travel, too. Dinner is then something light in the hotel coffee shop.

There is another sly move you can make when you find yourself in a place where the food is rather suspicious or unappetizing or both. What you do is order breakfast, no matter what the time of day. Almost every American greasy spoon, in even the smallest of towns, can produce good identifiable breakfast fare. You also see "breakfast served all day" on an increasing number of menus. (You'll also get somewhat of a reputation if you blink sleepily at them at noon or five o'clock and order breakfast, implying that you just got up after a wild night.)

Do I have to exercise? _____

A better question would be, "Isn't it terrific that such an enjoyable activity as exercise is a basic part of diabetes therapy?" The answer to both questions is yes.

Although exercise is often a neglected area in diabetes care, getting the right amount of exercise is just as important as following a good eating plan—if not more important.

We've heard it said that if you had to make a choice between eating junk food and exercising or eating a perfectly healthy diet and being immobile, you'd be healthier eating the junk food and exercising. Of course, a diabetic doesn't have to make that choice—in fact, can't make it. You need both exercise and good food for optimum health and blood sugar control.

Exercise is almost a magic formula for diabetics. If you're too thin—usually the lean insulin-dependent types—it will help you gain needed pounds by causing you to utilize your food better. Since it acts like an "invisible insulin," it helps get glucose into the cells, so less of it is wasted by being spilled into the urine.

If you're overweight, exercise will help you lose weight—and keep it off. Contrary to the myth, exercise does *not* increase your appetite. In fact, it suppresses it by regulating your *appestat,* the brain center that controls the appetite, and redirecting the blood flow away from the digestive tract. As a result, you'll be able to eat more because of the calories you burn, and yet you'll feel like eating less. This combination will deliver you from that complaint of so many diabetics: "I'm always hungry."

Besides helping overweight, non-insulin-dependent diabetics lose weight, exercise is now believed to lower your blood sugar by actually increasing the number of insulin receptors—those cell "locks" that the key of insulin is inserted into.

Exercise helps all diabetics improve circulation and lower blood fats (*cholesterol* and *triglycerides*) and therefore helps ward off the heart and blood vessel problems to which diabetics are subject.

What kind of exercise should I do?

What kind of exercise do you like? Exercise should be fun. That's the only way to be sure you'll keep doing it. As a diabetic you have enough chores in your life without turning exercise into another one.

If you want to rate exercises, though, the ones that are best for you are the aerobic or endurance kind: brisk walking, jogging, running, swimming, cross-country skiing, biking (either on the real thing or in bad weather on an exercycle), rowing, jumping rope. Dancing is also a wonderful endurance exercise. There are now even some special aerobic dance classes designed especially to build up your cardiovascular system and endurance.

But really, as we said, exercise is play and should be fun. Try to acquire a skill you enjoy like tennis or bowling or golf, even if it isn't an endurance sport. We find that if you get really involved in a nonendurance sport, you tend to do some endurance exercising in order to—what else?—increase your endurance for the sport you love.

Yoga is also a wonderful exercise to keep you supple, and it's something that can be done at any age.

Incidentally, don't let age stop you. Almost everyone can at least start walking and increase the distance and speed each day until it becomes the kind of endurance exercise that you need. Aim at first for a twenty-minute mile. If you attain that, then work toward a vigorous twelve-minute mile, which is right up there with jogging and running as far as conditioning is concerned.

As well as getting into a sport, it's important to bring more exercise into your daily life simply by becoming a more physically active person. Get up out of your chair and move whenever possible. Climb stairs rather than taking the elevator. Park your car in the farthest corner of the parking lot and walk to the store. (Since everybody else is always trying to get as close as possible, you'll get the dividend of not having your car dinged up by other people opening their doors on it.)

How about calisthenics?

If you like them, fine, but most people find them deadly dull, and anything you find deadly dull you're not likely to do for very long.

One kind of exercise that is *not* recommended is the isometrics. Those are the ones in which you pit one muscle against another. (Remember Charles Atlas and the old Dynamic Tension?) Doing this can put a strain on the heart. And they're no fun anyway.

How can I tell if my diabetes is in control?

You make tests. There are three kinds of tests you can make in your own home. We'll list them the way some mail-order catalogs list their products: good, better, best.

Good—urine testing

For years this has been the way most diabetics have checked on how well they were managing their diabetes. You test the amount of sugar in your urine. If you have no sugar, then the assumption is that your blood sugar has remained normal, because if it hadn't, sugar would have spilled over into your urine.

If there *is* sugar, the assumption is that your blood sugar was above normal at some time during the previous hours. The test shows the amount of sugar and this is supposed to indicate how high your blood sugar was—and may still be.

Urine testing for insulin-dependent diabetics is usually recommended four times a day—before meals and at bedtime. Other diabetics can often get by on one test two hours after the largest meal of the day.

There are three products you can use for urine testing:

1. Clinitest. These are little tablets you put in a test tube. You collect a specimen of urine and put in two or five drops (there are two methods to choose from) with an eyedropper. You add ten drops of water. Then you drop in a tablet. After the liquid finishes boiling, you wait fifteen seconds before comparing the color with a chart. The color remains dark blue (negative) or changes to green or gold or orange, depending on the percentage of sugar in the urine. If during the fifteen-second wait the color passes through the entire spectrum and ends up a dark greenish brown, the percentage of sugar is greater than the test can measure. The two-drop method is more accurate for higher ranges of blood sugar.

Clinitest is the most troublesome but also the most accurate way to test for sugar in your urine. It is most often recommended for insulin-dependent diabetics (the two-drop method).

2. Diastix. These are plastic sticks with a chemical testing area at the end. You can either dip the stick into a sample of urine or hold it in the stream of urine. Wait thirty seconds and compare the color of the stick tip with the color blocks on the container. The colors change from aqua (negative) to brown.

3. Tes-Tape. This is a roll of chemically treated tape. You tear off a piece and either dip it into a urine specimen or hold it in the stream. In one minute the strip either stays yellow (negative) or it changes to darkening shades of green, depending on the amount of sugar in the urine. If it stops at one-half percent (3+) at the end of this minute, then wait another minute before deciding on the amount of sugar.

The advantages of urine testing are its relatively low cost and its convenience. It's by far the least expensive of the testing methods. With Diastix and Tes-Tape you can make the tests quickly and easily whenever you're in a restroom.

The disadvantages of urine testing are several. The testing materials can give inaccurate results if affected by moisture or certain drugs you may be taking, such as vitamin C, some types of antibiotics, and aspirin. Even the amount of water you've been drinking can affect the reading. If you've been drinking a lot of water, the percetage of sugar in the urine will appear to be less than it really is.

Also remember that we said that many people, especially older people, have a high renal threshold. Their blood sugar has to be extremely high before the kidneys let sugar spill into their urine and register on a urine test. Conversely, children often have a very low threshold, and it looks as if they have very high blood sugar, when actually it's only slightly high or even normal.

Another main problem with urine tests is that they can only tell you if your blood sugar is high. If no sugar shows on a urine test, you don't know if your blood sugar is normal or low. With insulin-dependent diabetics it's just as important to know if blood sugar is too low as it is to know if it's too high.

As a matter of fact, urine testing doesn't even show you what your blood sugar is at the moment that you make the test. If you have a positive test for sugar, you only know that your blood sugar *was* high. You only know past history. Naturally, it's good to know whether you've been in control or not, but, especially for insulin takers, the information can be deceptive and dangerous. They might assume their blood sugar is high after a positive urine test, when in reality it could have already fallen low and they could need to eat something to bring it up.

Some doctors and nurses believe that if you take what's called a second void, the urine test is more accurate. A second void means you urinate once without testing and then half an hour later you urinate again and do the test from that. This test usually reflects blood sugar one-half to one hour before. Recent studies, however, have somewhat discredited this theory. They show that accuracy is improved very little, if at all, by the second-void method.

Another disadvantage of urine testing is that people don't enjoy fiddling around with their urine. It's just not an aesthetically pleasing activity and some diabetics find it positively degrading. At best, you have to keep your sense of humor operative.

Better—home blood sugar testing with Chemstrips bG or Dextrostix

The new, improved way of finding out if you're in control is by testing your blood sugar. The advantage of accuracy in this is obvious: The test tells if your blood sugar *itself* is low or normal or high, and it tells you what it is at the very moment you take it. As San Francisco diabetologist Dr. Alan Rubin says, it's the difference between a person and the shadow of a person. The blood sugar test is the person, the urine test merely a shadow.

We ourselves are more enthusiastic about home blood sugar testing than we are about any recent development in diabetes care. We agree totally with Dr. Donnell Etzwiler, Director of the Diabetes Education Center in Minneapolis, Minnesota, who considers home blood sugar testing such an important tool in the management of diabetes that ". . . we can anticipate that perhaps by 1985 urine testing by diabetic patients will be a thing of the past."

Previously the only way you could have a blood sugar test was in a doctor's office or hospital. Now it's possible to do it at home by pricking your finger to get a drop of blood and putting it on a chemical agent at the end of a stick. You read the results by matching the color on the end of the stick to a color chart printed on the side of the container of the sticks. The two kinds of sticks currently available for this purpose are Chemstrips bG and Dextrostix. Chemstrips bG (Figure 1) are

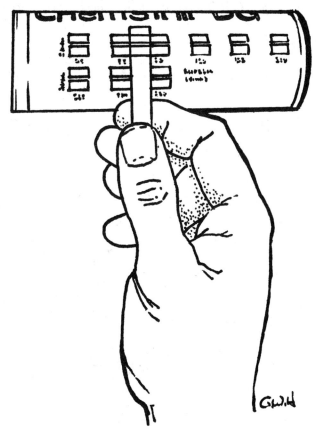

FIGURE 1   CHEMSTRIPS bG

easier to read since they have two colors to match (beige and turquoise) instead of just one; and Chemstrips bG, unlike Dextrostix, are wiped off with cotton instead of being rinsed with water so you can test yourself anywhere. (June has done it sitting in an airplane or riding as a passenger in a car.)

You can easily see one of the disadvantages of testing your blood sugar—getting the drop of blood from your finger. Nobody likes to jab a finger with a needle or one of those little bloodletting blades called lancets. Fortunately, there is a new device to help get the blood. It's called the Autolet (Figure 2). Using it, you can press a button and automatically and almost painlessly get the sample of blood you need.

Another disadvantage to home blood sugar testing is the cost. As of this writing Autolets cost $25.00 and each time you use a stick it currently costs between forty-two cents and seventy-five cents, depending on where you buy them. And even at high prices, it's not always easy to find blood sugar testing sticks and Autolets. (If your pharmacy doesn't stock them, they are available from the Sugarfree Center.)

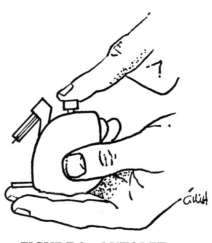

FIGURE 2   AUTOLET

It's also difficult for some diabetics, especially those with vision problems, to read the colors accurately. (With Chemstrips bG we suggest you judge primarily by the bottom color, turquoise, for below normal blood sugars and by the top color, beige, for above normal blood sugars because it is easier to distinguish the variations in those colors in those ranges.) Generally, however, you have no problem deciding whether your blood sugar is low or high or in the normal range, and that's usually enough to know. If you need to know your *exact* blood sugar, say within five or ten points of accuracy, you have to use the *best* way of testing.

Best—home blood sugar testing with sticks and a meter

It's possible to buy a meter into which you insert a stick after putting a blood sample on it. The meter then gives you a specific readout, the kind you formerly could only get by going to your doctor's office or a hospital laboratory.

With a meter you can know exactly what your blood sugar is at any given moment and you can gear your management plan to the facts rather than to guesswork. For pregnant diabetics, for diabetics with high or low urine thresholds, and for insulin-dependent diabetics who have mysterious swings of blood sugar, or, as a matter of fact, for any diabetic, the meter can make the difference between feeling good and feeling bad, between feeling defeated and feeling victorious, and as more and more doctors are coming to believe, between developing complications and being free of them.

The meters now available are manufactured by the same firms that market the sticks, the Ames Company of Elkhart, Indiana and Bio-Dynamics of Indianapolis, Indiana. There are now three generations of meters in the Ames family but still only one in the Bio-Dynamics family.

Ames meters

Eyetone reflectance colorimeter. This is the first generation and the one that June first owned. It weighs 2¾ pounds
and measures 7¼ inches long, 4½ inches wide, and 2 inches
high. This machine served June well. Though plugged into the
electricity for over two years, it was still going strong when
June switched to a later model.

Different bottles of Dextrostix have slight variations in
how they react to the blood sample, so for accuracy, each time
a new bottle is opened, the machine must be calibrated (ad-
justed) to that particular bottle of sticks. A simplified and accurate way to calibrate it is described in Richard K. Bernstein's
book, *Diabetes: The Glucograf Method for Normalizing Blood Sugar*
(see Suggested Reading). The Eyetone is no longer being manufactured, but you may be able to locate a used one through
your Ames representative or an individual, and at a price con-
siderably less than the later models.

Dextrometer. This is the second generation and the machine that is currently on the market. It weighs 13½ ounces
and measures 6¼ inches long, 3⅛ inches wide, and 1½ inches
high. It has a battery pack, which allows you to carry it with
you and use it when you're away from home. The problem
with using it on batteries is that it must be calibrated each time
you turn it on. This means using two Dextrostix for each
blood sugar you take. If you keep it plugged into the electricity, this disadvantage is overcome. The Dextrometer costs
$275; the battery pack is $35 extra. (See Figure 3.)

Glucometer. This, the third generation, is now available
only in England, but will be coming onto the American market in 1982. It is only 3¼ inches long, 6⅝ inches wide and
15/6 inches high and weighs 12 ounces with batteries. (It oper-
ates only on batteries; you can't plug it in.) You can carry it in

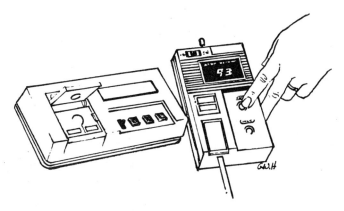

FIGURE 3   GLUCOMETER AND DEXTROMETER

an overcoat pocket or a purse. And best of all, it can store its calibration in its memory even when turned off. (See Figure 3.)

According to an Ames representative we talked with, the Glucometer is the first meter truly designed with the diabetic in mind instead of laboratories and doctors' offices. June has been using an English model of it and considers it a marvel. It beeps to tell you when to put your drop of blood on the strip and beeps again to tell you when to wash it off. It's such a perfect gem of a little machine that she thinks she'd like to marry it. In fact, in a sense she already has.

We'll let a diabetic laboratory technician we know, Dixie Starkovich of Redondo Beach, California, have the final word on blood sugar testing. Dixie did a comparison of home blood sugar monitoring methods. She took thirty blood sugars using Chemstrips bG and compared her results with readings on a Dextrometer, a StatTek meter, and the Coulter serum blood testing method used by laboratories.

Dixie told us that she is extremely impressed with how accurate and close to each other all methods of checking blood sugar are. Her conclusion is that if you have good color vision, you can do just as well with Chemstrips bG as with meters. You have to remember, of course, that Dixie has a laboratory-trained eye for reading color changes. She also has scientific objectivity. Some diabetics, when dealing with their own blood sugar, tend to invariably read Chemstrips bG higher or lower than they really are, either out of worry or wishful thinking.

Bio-dynamics meter

StatTek. This meter is made by the same firm that makes Chemstrips bG, but it cannot give readings from them. Special strips called "StatTek glucose test strips" are required.

The StatTek has been used by laboratories for many years, but only recently was its price lowered enough to put it in competition with the Ames meters. It now costs $375. It weighs 2¼ pounds and is 8½ inches long, 5¾ inches wide, and 4 inches high. There is no battery pack available. Calibration is simple, but without a special adapter kit the meter only registers blood sugar from 40 to 350. (The Ames meters register 0 to 400.)

We have heard that Bio-Dynamics is about to burst onto the scene with a new machine comparable to the Glucometer. Watch for it.

What June does is test her blood sugar with her meter at home; she uses Chemstrips bG without the meter when she's away from home. That way she has the best of both worlds.

How often should you test your blood sugar at home?

Some doctors recommend blood sugar testing as few as four times a week; others advise doing it as often as four times a day (or more!). June usually does hers twice a day—before breakfast and when she gets home from work in the late afternoon. She also does it when she's confused about what her blood sugar is because she's having trouble reading her body signals. This can be pretty often when she's under pressure or on a trip or doing an extra lot of exercising or is otherwise out of her regular routines. Many diabetics like to test two hours after eating to see how they handled the meal.

Richard K. Bernstein, who advocates very tight control for juvenile diabetics, has evolved a system called "Glucograf." In this system, diabetics test as frequently as six times a day in order to keep their blood sugar normal 90 percent of the time and thereby avoid the complications long-term juvenile diabetics can be susceptible to. His book, *Diabetes: The Glucograf Method for Normalizing Blood Sugar*, describes this system (see Suggested Reading).

Do you ever need to go to the doctor for tests if you do them yourself at home?

Yes, you should go about every three months for a *glycohemoglobin test* (hemoglobin A_{lc}). This is a new test that reveals the amount of glucose clinging to individual cells. It tells you how your overall control has been over a 100-day period.

The glycohemoglobin test is a great improvement over going to the doctor for a simple blood sugar test because it doesn't really allow you to fool yourself or your doctor. We are all only human and we want the doctor to think well of us. We want to be patted on the back for being the well-behaved patients we should be. Consequently, we tend to be much more meticulous about diabetes care immediately before visiting the doctor for a blood sugar. The hemoglobin A_{lc} reveals whether you've been taking care of your diabetes all the time, rather than just the two or three hours prior to your visit to the doctor.

Are there any other tests that I need to know about?

Yes, there is one more important one: testing for ketones. You'll remember that ketones are the substances that accumulate in the blood and subsequently the urine, when glucose isn't getting into the cells and you're having to burn your own fat and muscle for fuel.

Several years ago there was a fad diet that had people eating only protein and fat (no carbohydrate). They were to test their urine for ketones every day and to be happy when they found ketones in it, because that meant they were burning fat and therefore losing weight.

Diabetics should *not* be happy to find ketones in their urine. In fact, if you should find them along with 2 percent or over sugar, contact your doctor *immediately* for advice on how to get rid of them. This combination means you are seriously out of control.

How do I test for ketones?

A better question might be, *when* do I test for ketones? The answer for diabetics on insulin is whenever two consecutive urine tests measure 2 percent sugar or when your blood sugar tests are over 200. For non-insulin-dependent diabetics who still produce some insulin of their own, the situation is not so crucial. Those who have a high renal threshold and are running higher blood sugar than they realize, can, of course get in trouble. (See why it's important to know your renal threshold?) All diabetics need to watch for ketones when they have infections or illnesses or out-of-the-ordinary emotional stress.

Now, how do you test? There are two products to use:

Ketostix. This is a stick. You dip it into urine, wait fifteen seconds, and compare with six color blocks to determine the amount of ketones. (Keto-Diastix measure both ketones and glucose on the same stick.)

Acetest. This is a tablet. You place a drop of urine on it, wait thirty seconds, and then compare the result with a color chart.

Since urine and blood sugar and ketone tests are important information for your doctor as well as for you, it's smart to keep a written record of your tests. For this purpose the Ames Company has published an attractive compact daily diary called *Clinilog*, which also contains a lot of valuable reference information. They'll send you a copy for $1.00. (Write to Dept. JRP, Ames Company, Division Miles Laboratories, Inc., Elkhart, Indiana 46514.)

Richard K. Bernstein has designed the Glucograf, a printed form for charting your injections, blood sugars, meal, exercise, in fact your entire diabetes regimen. It's available from the Sugarfree Center in pads of 52, one for each week of the year.

Since I don't take insulin, do I have to do all of that urine and blood sugar testing?

Absolutely. Even though you don't generally have a problem with low blood sugar, you do have one with high blood sugar. As you know, it's the high blood sugar that causes the damage. You have to know when it's high, so you can do something to bring it down—exercise, change your diet, etc.

When we first learned about home blood sugar testing, we thought it wouldn't be necessary for non-insulin-dependent diabetics. Urine tests, we thought, would do the job for them. We've since changed our minds.

Home blood sugar testing is equally important for non-insulin-takers. Most are older when they're diagnosed, and re member, the older you get, the higher goes your renal threshold.

You might take a urine test when your blood sugar is, say, 215, and the test will tell you that your blood sugar is normal when in reality it's dangerously high.

For example, we talked to the daugher of a diabetic woman who, according to her daughter, "*loves* to eat, especially at big family gatherings." The mother would take her urine test, it would show that she wasn't spilling sugar, so presuming her blood sugar to be normal, she'd sit down happily and, as her daughter put it, "have a feast."

The woman wound up in the hospital with dangerous ketoacidosis. She'd been running extremely high blood sugar, but it had never shown up in her urine test because of her high renal threshold.

This woman is now testing her blood sugar regularly at home. She doesn't have many feasts these days, but she's going to be around for a lot more regular meals than she would have been had she continued to dwell in a diabetic's fool's paradise with her urine tests.

Another insidious aspect about being casual with your self-care and testing is that if you run around too long with elevated blood sugar, diabetes complications can start slowly and quietly developing. You may never even know what is going on until the damage is done. We're not fear-mongers and we don't like to threaten you with the problems diabetics are heir to, but in our experience, non-insulin-dependent diabetics don't get the point about the seriousness of diabetes the way insulin takers do.

Remember that, even if you don't take insulin, you have to be as careful as any other diabetic. Actually non-insulin-takers are the most likely candidates for arrival at the hospital with diabetes-related complications or, as diabetes nurse specialist Diana Guthrie warns, "to have to have part of a leg removed," because they're the ones most likely to ignore their diabetes until it screams for attention.

What should I expect from my doctor?

You should expect your doctor to schedule you for regular visits every two to three months—maybe at times as frequently as every week or so. She or he will probably order laboratory tests—blood sugars or glycohemoglobins, for example—to keep you informed on how well you're doing and to be able to help you assess your routines and advise you on any changes needed. Your doctor should also be available by telephone (or have a colleague who is available) at all times in case any serious diabetes-related emergency develops and you need help. The doctor should be willing to answer occasional questions by phone when you're having trouble handling some diabetes problem.

All this is just standard care, however. The more important expectations you should have deal with your doctor's attitude and your interaction with him or her.

First and foremost, you should expect your doctor to treat you as an individual, not just a textbook diabetes case. You are a person with definite needs and interests and likes and dislikes and they can and should be incorporated into your treatment. There are many different ways of handling diabetes—different diets, different exercise plans, even different insulin injection schedules that can make diabetes come at least halfway toward adjusting to your lifestyle.

In order for the doctor to make these variations on the basic theme of diabetes care, she or he is going to have to spend a little time finding out about you and your way of living, working, and playing. In other words, your doctor is going to have to talk to you. No, make that talk *with* you. There should be an interchange of ideas, not a lecture. The doctor should regard you as a colleague in your diabetes care and never convey the idea that you are incapable of understanding your condition and treatment. In fact, as Dr. Donnell B. Etzwiler says,

"Diabetic patients provide 99 percent of their own care." So as your own physician you'd *better* be capable of understanding your condition and its treatment.

Your doctor, therefore, should give you a full explanation of all the laboratory tests you have. Rather than telling you your blood sugar is "normal" or "a little high, but still okay," he or she should tell you the exact figures. You should also know exactly where you stand with cholesterol, triglycerides, blood pressure, everything that affects your health and that you can make better or worse by your own behavior.

Now although there are a lot of things that your doctor has to discuss with you, we don't want to lead you to expect that the doctor should have long, leisurely conversations with you, going over every facet of your physiological and psychological makeup. A doctor's time is too valuable to squander in great chunks. You are not the only patient and others have their needs, too.

And speaking of time, *your* time has some value too. You deserve a doctor who doesn't overbook and keep patients crouching in the waiting room for hours, building up stresses that are very bad for diabetes control.

This is not to say you should *never* have to wait. There are emergencies that a doctor must handle and they can throw the schedule off, but if there is an emergency every time you have an appointment, you have cause for suspicion. We wouldn't carry on about waiting time to this extent except that since a diabetic goes to the doctor regularly every two or three months *forever*, that waiting room time can really add up.

Since most doctors frankly admit that they lack a background in nutrition—one doctor told us he had had only a one-hour lecture on it during his entire time at medical school—you should expect your doctor to be able to refer you to a good dietitian to help you plan the complexities and personal variations of your diet. He or she shouldn't just throw a one-page diet list at you and send you on your way.

It is also extremely helpful if the office has a diabetes nurse specialist who can help you develop a good technique with injections, blood sugar and urine testing, diet, and problems of daily living. Again, these are specifics that the doctor doesn't have the time to help you with.

You should expect your doctor to keep up with the latest developments in the field of diabetes and be willing to incorporate them into your treatment. New developments—such as home blood sugar testing—usually bring a lot more flexibility to your diabetes program and help you maintain general good health.

Finally—and this may be asking too much—we personally feel that your doctor and other involved health professionals should also provide a good example. It's rather difficult for you to take good health advice from a flabby chain-smoker who is obviously ignoring all such counsel. June's doctor is as lean as she is and he and she have cholesterol races to see who can get it the lowest. Despite the fact that men generally have higher cholesterol, at the moment he's winning by two points. Incidentally, if your doctor is one of these paragons of medical virtue, please write and tell us his or her name. Diabetics sometimes ask us for recommendations.

From all these "shoulds," you can see that it helps a great deal if your doctor is a diabetologist or an internist who specializes in diabetes.

How do I find a doctor who specializes in diabetes?

Call your local diabetes association and ask them for the names of diabetologists who are closest to your home (and closeness *is* important). If your town has no local association, call your state affiliate of the American Diabetes Association and ask them for a recommendation.

If you still have no luck, call your local hospital and ask who on their staff handles most of the diabetes cases.

Another good thing to do is go to your public library and check the *Directory of Medical Specialists* (see Suggested Reading). This way you can find out the doctor's training, what hospitals he or she has worked in, age, and special experience.

We realize, however, that in some small towns there simply isn't a diabetologist. In that case, find (or keep) a doctor with whom you feel you can have a good relationship. Look for one who is willing to explore solutions to problems you present. Be sure she or he is willing to investigate new developments in diabetes that you may learn about in your reading or from discussions at meetings and seminars.

Incidentally, if you have a beloved family doctor, there's no reason to desert him or her for a diabetologist. You can keep the beloved one as your general physician and go to your diabetologist for specific diabetes care.

When your diabetes is in its early stages or if you start developing problems at any time, you may want to go to one of the major diabetes clinics in the country where you stay a week or so and they give you examinations and lab tests. You attend classes and learn what you need to do to get your diabetes in good control.

After all this talk about what your doctor should do for you, we mustn't forget your responsibilities to your doctor and what your doctor should expect from you.

What should my doctor expect from me?

Number one is honesty. Always tell the doctor the truth about what you're doing (or not doing) in your diabetes care. Report the true results of your urine and blood sugar tests. (One young woman told us she faked the results of the tests because she didn't want the doctor to be disappointed!) The doctor can't get you on the right track if he or she doesn't know that you're on the wrong one. Never try to fake the doctor out by behaving like a model diabetic for the few days just before you're scheduled for an examination and being very casual (sloppy) about your self-care the rest of the time.

You also owe your doctor cooperation. If you can't or won't follow the advice you're given, you should find another doctor whose advice you can and will accept.

Your doctor should also be able to expect you to take good care of yourself—not just your diabetes, but your *whole self.* Too many of us think we can neglect our health or even actively destroy it and then go to the doctor and say, "I'm sick. Make me well." Then if the doctor can't rectify the damage we've done, we get angry. We like the medical policy that they have in Germany. Government health insurance won't pay for physical problems brought on by smoking. They believe that if you deliberately abuse your body in that way, you should be the one to pay the consequences—and the bill.

Don't take advantage of your doctor. If you phone constantly to discuss every little problem, try to monopolize his or her time in the office, using the doctor as a father or mother confessor, you're actually taking advantage of other patients whose time you're usurping.

It's ironic, but once you've found a doctor who is willing to listen, you have to be responsible enough to restrain yourself and stick to the facts of your diabetes problem. Your personal life problems *are* a part of the total picture of your diabetes, true, but a mention of their existence is enough. A diabetologist is not a psychiatrist and cannot be expected to straighten out your marriage, assuage your guilt feelings, release your inhibitions or do whatever else is required to give you psychic peace.

If your life problems weigh unbearably upon you and you feel they are significantly detrimental to your diabetes control, then ask your diabetologist to recommend a therapist to help you with them.

How can I learn more about taking care of my diabetes? _____

Read books, read periodicals like *Diabetes Forecast, Diabetes in the News*, and, if you have a scientific turn of mind, *Diabetes Care* (see Suggested Reading). Skip *Diabetes Outlook*. It's mainly for doctors and, besides, those Grand Guignol, full-color illustrations of gangrenous toes which they like to feature don't do much for fostering an optimistic attitude.

Join your local affiliate of the American Diabetes Association (see Reference Section: Directory of Services for Diabetics) and attend their meetings. They usually have a guest speaker—a podiatrist, dietitian, ophthalmologist, or some such person, who can fill you in on their own areas of expertise and answer questions that may have been puzzling you. Diabetes associations often sponsor day-long seminars with different speakers, panel discussions, and workshops. These are a terrific way to get a lot of diabetes information in a short period of time.

Find a diabetes education program in your area. Ask the ADA for names and places or write to the American Association of Diabetes Educators (see Reference Section: Directory of Services for Diabetics). These education programs sometimes charge a nominal fee, but you always get a lot more than your money's worth. Besides, many health insurance companies are starting to reimburse you for diabetes education programs— and well they should, since these programs do a lot toward helping you stay healthy and thereby saving the companies money in the long run.

Diabetes education programs can be a one-week crash course or weekly meetings over a period of time. They can be inpatient programs for newly diagnosed diabetics in the hospital, but most are outpatient. The groups can be large or small or they can be individual instruction. There may be a group of teachers (nurses, dietitians, psychologists, social workers, etc.) or there may be one diabetes educator who handles the whole course. As you can see, you can usually find a program to meet your needs whatever those needs may be.

Some diabetics we know are starting to form their own discussion groups so they can share experiences and helpful information with each other. Your doctor or the diabetes association or a diabetes education program may be able to put you in touch with other diabetics who are interested in forming such a group. You'll especially want to join a group if you agree with diabetic author Dorothea Sims: "Loneliness is one of the hardest things about having diabetes." (See Reference Section: Suggested Readings.)

Speaking of discussion groups, a film that we particularly recommend is "Diabetes: Focus on Feelings." It shows a discussion group led by UCLA Diabetes Educator and Clinical Social Work Consultant, Noreen Hall Papatheodorou. This is a tremendously moving and revealing film that can crack the shell of the most resentful and intractable of diabetics and can give family members insights into a diabetic's feelings that might otherwise take years to pry out. Ms. Papatheodorou has written a discussion guide to go with the film, and both are available from Pyramid Films, Box 1048, Santa Monica, California 90406. You might write to them and ask if the film is scheduled for showing in your area. If not, you could get together with a group and rent it yourself.

Keep at your learning. It's not just a one-time thing. There are new things to learn every day and the new things almost invariably improve your health and make your life as a diabetic easier to handle.

Should I tell people I have diabetes?

In general, definitely yes. You should tell everyone you have any kind of everyday contact with—your hairdresser or barber, your colleagues at work, your teachers, your coaches, your friends, even rather casual ones, and especially those with whom you play sports.

You should make it a special point to tell anyone with whom you have any kind of medical or semi-medical dealings, such as your dentist or podiatrist or oculist, because that may influence their treatment of you.

There are several good reasons for letting people know you have diabetes, especially if you are insulin-dependent. In the first place, should you have an insulin reaction, a person in the know can help you out or at least will realize that whatever is happening to you may be related to your diabetes and will get you to someone who can help.

You are also much less likely to inadvertently offend people if they know you have diabetes. For example, if you get low blood sugar and suddenly turn into a grouch or hellion, they may realize it's because of your diabetes, not because of a mean streak that's part of your nature. Then, too, if you're eating at a friend's house and turn down a sugar-shot confection, the cook will know that you're not insulting his or her talents but just behaving yourself and following your diabetic diet.

Another reason for informing on your diabetes is that you can help out other diabetics by educating nondiabetics as to what diabetes is. What diabetics need is an each-one-teach-one program in order to spread diabetes facts and wipe out some of those weird fictions that are floating around in the public mind, such as "Diabetics can't eat sugar, but they can eat all the honey they want because honey is natural."

If you do tell others about your diabetes, you're also likely to gain a lot of diabetic friends. That is to say, a number of people you already know will come out of the closet and declare themselves when you confess your "guilty secret."

When June was first diagnosed, she was such a babe-in-the-woods that she didn't know that a lot of people hid their diabetes, as if it were a social disease rather than a metabolic one. She just blurted it out to everyone. To her amazement, it turned out that she knew five diabetics when she thought she didn't know any.

Later, June went through a period of diabetic self-consciousness and started covering up. That didn't last long. Barbara was always on the job spreading the news loud and clear. Every time we flew in an airplane, for example, Barbara informed the flight attendant of June's condition and announced to the person occupying the third seat in our row, "My friend here has diabetes. Before lunch is served, I'm going to be giving her an insulin shot. I hope it won't bother you, but if it does, you can look the other way."

That used to make June cringe, but now in thinking back on it, she admits it was a good idea. After all, who knows what our seatmate might have thought was going on with that needle? And if June should need a quick snack, the flight attendant would be alerted and would supply it fast and without question. Also, it helped her accept the fact that she has diabetes and not develop any psychological hang-ups about it.

As part of your diabetes announcement program, you should certainly wear some sort of identification bracelet or medallion. This is a safeguard in case you are ever in an accident or have some sort of diabetic problem when you're away from those who know you. A particularly good identification is a Medic Alert bracelet. (This is available from Medic Alert Foundation, P. O. Box 1009, Turlock, California 95380, phone 209-632-2371.) Medic Alert is well known now, and ambulance attendants and members of the ski patrol and doctors and nurses in emergency hospitals are on the lookout for their insignia. June wears her Medic Alert bracelet always, even when she's asleep.

Now, after advocating this policy of extreme honesty, we'll hedge a bit. You don't have to be obsessed with your diabetes and immediately tell everyone you meet, "Hello-there-I'm-John-Smith-and-I'm-a-diabetic-pleased-to-meet-you," any more than you'd announce to a new acquaintance that you have gallstones or are color-blind or wear a pacemaker. As you get to know people better, your diabetes will emerge appropriately and naturally as a subject for conversation.

As for telling prospective employers and insurance agents, it's a yes and no situation that we'll discuss in those sections.

Which is the correct thing to say: "I am a diabetic," or "I have diabetes?"

Either is correct. It's a matter of personal preference. *Diabetes in the News* once ran a reader survey to see which way most diabetics like it better. "I am a diabetic" won a clear victory. Most people thought it was more straightforward and more accepting of your condition.

A case can be made, however, for "I have diabetes." It sounds more as if you are giving yourself primary importance and your disease only secondary importance. You're a person who just happens to have diabetes.

Either of these phrases will make you easily understood. Don't shy away from them and use something cryptic the way June did once on a flight to Hawaii, when she was trying to get her meal from the flight attendant. "I'm on insulin," she said. "Could you serve me first?" The answer was negative. The problem, we figured out later, was that the flight attendant, who was Danish, didn't have any idea what June was talking about. In fact, she probably thought that insulin was the name of some kind of group tour of the islands and that June was just trying to get a special privilege for no good reason.

When Barbara trotted back a few minutes later and made eyeball-to-eyeball contact with the flight attendant and announced, "My friend is a di-a-bet-ic and she needs to eat. Could you serve her now?" the meal appeared a few seconds faster than immediately.

Experts have very definite ideas about correctness, in the use of the words diabetes and diabetic. They don't like you to use diabetic as an adjective, unless what you're talking about actually has diabetes. For example, "The diabetic man had a diabetic dog," is all right, because both the man and the dog are diabetics. "The diabetic education lecture was held at the diabetic study center," is all wrong, because neither the education lecture nor the study center has diabetes. It should be, "The diabetes education lecture was held at the diabetes study center."

You wouldn't say "a diabetic specialist," unless the specialist you're talking about has diabetes. If he's a specialist in diabetes, he should be called a diabetes specialist. If he's a specialist in diabetes who has diabetes, then presumably he'd be referred to as a "diabetic diabetes specialist." But maybe you think this is being linguistically nit-picky. Maybe we think so, too; since, as you may notice, we often use the word "diabetic" in the unaccepted way, and, in fact, interchange "diabetic" and "diabetes" especially when referring to the diet.

Just to put the capper on the whole nomenclatural confusion, the British call their organization "The British Diabetic Association." But they always did have trouble with the language.

Will my diabetes cause sex problems?

That depends to a certain extent on whether you are a woman or a man. Previously it had been thought that diabetes had little or no effect on either a woman's sexual performance or satisfaction. Even now, based on what diabetic women report to their doctors, it would seem that they reach a sexual climax just as often as nondiabetic women.

Still there are rumblings from some diabetes therapists—especially female diabetes therapists—that sex problems associated with diabetes are as common among women as among men. It's just that the male sex problems have been given more attention. This is not necessarily due to sexism. It may be due to the fact that sexual response is easier to measure with men than with women.

The majority of women's sexual problems appear to be related to poor diabetes control. A woman understandably loses interest in sex when she is excessively tired and rundown from being out of control. High blood sugar and the resulting sugar in the urine increase susceptibility to vaginal infections that cause swelling, itching, burning, and pain, which are hardly conducive to enthusiasm for sexual intercourse. These infections can be treated with salves, but the only real cure is keeping your diabetes in control.

If a long-term diabetic woman develops neuropathy (damaged nerve cells)—again often as a result of poor control—it may involve the nerve fibers that stimulate the genitalia so that arousal may not occur, making intercourse painful because lubricating fluids are not released. Arthur Krosnick, M.D., writing in the September–October, 1980 *Diabetes Forecast*, recommends the use of water soluble lubricants, such as K-Y Lubricating Jelly for this condition. He also states that "Estrogen deficiency responds to vaginal creams. These creams are available by prescription and do not affect diabetes control."

Although emotional factors associated with diabetes—anxiety, fear, anger—can have some effect on a woman's sex life, blood sugar control appears to be far more significant.

As for men, there has been a lot of talk about diabetes causing impotence. There has been so much talk, in fact, that the resulting fear has been known to cause it. A psychologist we heard speak told about one of his patients who wasn't aware of the existence of diabetic impotence and was getting along just fine. When he did hear the discouraging word, it was instant impotence for him. (We hope we're not doing harm by making you aware of the problem.)

The impotence legends and actualities have been brought about by several factors. Sometimes when a man is an undiagnosed, out-of-control diabetic, he can develop a *temporary* impotence, which goes away when he gets in control.

Sometimes when diabetes is first diagnosed, a man is shot with so many negative emotions such as anxiety, depression, anger, guilt, and fear of rejection that he becomes impotent for psychological reasons.

Sometimes problems are caused by what sex therapists Masters and Johnson call "spectatoring." Raul C. Schiavi and Barbara Hogan, writing in the January–February, 1979 issue of *Diabetes Care,* vividly describe the situation: "The diabetic patient, rather than becoming involved in the sexual experience and abandoning himself into erotic sensations and feelings, may find himself constantly monitoring the state of his penis. He becomes a witness rather than a participant in the sexual experience."

Not surprisingly this "performance anxiety" often results in impotence. Indeed, the *British Medical Journal* reported that impotence was most likely caused by psychological factors in two-thirds of the men studied and by physical factors in only one-third.

The well-known broadcaster and syndicated columnist, Dr. Gabe Mirkin, has discovered an easy and inexpensive (especially if you use one-cent stamps) test to determine if impotence is psychological or physical.

He explains that "There are two stages of sleep: rapid eye movement (REM) and nonrapid eye movement sleep. In nonrapid eye movement sleep, males achieve an erection. This can occur several times throughout the night and the male wakes up the next morning without even knowing about it."

If you are achieving erections in the night, then your impotence is psychological. To check this out, Dr. Mirkin recommends taking a roll of postage stamps, tearing off the appropriate number of stamps (he suggests four), and securing them tightly to the penis before going to bed. If the stamps are torn apart in the morning, then you know you're having erections.

To make sure that anxiety resulting in fitful sleep doesn't confuse the issue, it might be an idea to try this test more than once before deciding that your impotence is physical rather than psychological.

Since this is obviously a test that June can't check out personally, we'd appreciate it if you could let us know if this test works.

What can you do about impotence that is mainly psychological?

We hope it will help some just to have the reassurance that it *is* mainly psychological and that when you start handling the negative emotions that engulfed you with your diagnosis of diabetes the sex problem will gradually disappear.

We know, however, that such emotions and their effects can't always be swept away with logic and Dutch uncle conversations with yourself. You can't immediately eliminate your problem just because you've been told what's causing it. It takes time and consideration (consideration of yourself by yourself as well as consideration from your partner). If it takes too much time—and only you can decide how much is too much—you shouldn't hesitate to get some psychological help.

If your doctor isn't able to recommend a psychological counselor or sex therapist, you can contact any large university in your area. Most of these have human sexuality programs and can give you the names of qualified sex therapists who are available for private consultation.

What about physical impotence in diabetic men?

Then it's usually a gradual, long-term process caused by nerve damage. This can often be prevented by good diabetes control. When it does develop, however, counseling with a qualified sex therapist is again in order. He or she can advise you on alternative ways of giving and experiencing sexual pleasure as well as help you decide if penile prosthesis would be a good solution to your problem.

There are two kinds of prosthesis currently available: the semirigid rod and the inflatable. Many men have had success with penile prosthesis, but it is not something you should rush into without careful consideration and without thoroughly discussing the idea with your sexual partner.

You can become impotent while under the influence of certain drugs. Among these are alcohol, tranquilizers, marijuana, estrogens, and drugs for hypertension. In many older men impotence may be caused by hypertension drugs with diabetes getting the blame. When possible these suspect drugs should be avoided or their use should be discontinued.

Richard K. Bernstein, in his book, *Diabetes: the Glucograf Method For Normalizing Blood Sugar,* offers some practical advice for insulin-dependent diabetics. He explains that "inability to become aroused or if aroused inability to achieve orgasm, can be an early warning of hypoglycemia. . . . This early warning sign has been detected by both males and females. In fact, patients have located the [blood sugar levels] at which they 'turn off.'" He says, "It appears that both men and women tend to have two turn off points—at one [blood sugar level] they can be aroused but cannot achieve orgasm. At a lower [blood sugar level] they cannot even be aroused . . . Some patients try to prevent an unpleasant situation by measuring [blood sugar] (when feasible) prior to anticipated intercourse and promptly take fast acting sweets if blood sugar is low."

If you have some unanswered questions on the subject of impotence and if you have a fair understanding of medical terminology, ask your hospital librarian to let you read the January–February, 1979 issue of *Diabetes Care*, which is devoted to the subject of Sex and Diabetes.

Does diabetes cause male sterility?

No. Studies have shown that it does not affect your sperm count.

Should I become pregnant? _____

We assume from this question that you have already wrestled through the basic Everywoman life decision of whether or not to have children and have concluded that you want to, but you worry about the effect your diabetes will have on your baby and vice versa.

If that is the case, then the first step is to consult both your diabetologist (or internist or family doctor) and a gynecologist to see if there is any physical reason why pregnancy would be a poor risk for you.

If their reaction is positive, then you can be cheered by the news that the death rate of babies of diabetic mothers has been significantly reduced in the past ten years and is now closer to that of the general population. Both mother and child come through successfully more than 90 percent of the time.

To improve your odds even further you should heed the advice of Dr. Edith Miller of the Joslin Clinic (*Diabetes Forecast* March–April, 1980) who says that diabetic women who want to have children should be in the best possible control *before* becoming pregnant (have a hemoglobin A_{1c} test to find out) and stay in good control from the time of conception on.

This advice is backed up by a study of the pregnancies of twenty-five women that was reported in the *British Medical Journal*. These women had previously had fourteen pregnancies among them. Out of these fourteen pregnancies, six babies had been lost either during pregnancy or soon after birth. For this study the women were all put on home blood sugar monitoring. Result: the women were not only able to maintain good blood sugar level, but *every one delivered a healthy baby.*

For a very brittle diabetic it may also be wise to go onto the pump during pregnancy (see For Insulin-Dependent Diabetics: What Is this Insulin Pump I'm Hearing So Much About?).

We find it hard to conceive of the idea that health insurance, if you have it, would not pay for all the costs of blood sugar monitoring and, if necessary, the pump during pregnancy. It would be a sound investment on their part since the alternative could be astronomical hospital bills (in the $25,000 range).

We find it impossible to conceive of the idea that your doctor wouldn't want you to do home blood sugar monitoring, either alone or in conjunction with a pump, during your pregnancy.

If your main decision on whether or not to have a baby involves the ethics of producing a child with the possibility of diabetic heredity, than that's a decision only you can make. Since the pattern of inheritance of diabetes is unclear, each family must make a personal assessment of risks of having diabetic children. You can get counseling by requesting it through your diabetes educator or by contacting your nearest chapter of the National Foundation March of Dimes and asking for their list of genetic centers and genetic services.

While deciding, you might consider the fact that every human being carries many defective genes and having a baby involves playing genetic lottery. You might also ask yourself if you'd prefer to have been born programmed for diabetes or not to have been born at all.

On the other hand, many diabetic women and their mates ultimately decide to adopt a child. It occurred to us that since there's currently a shortage of "perfect" babies available for adoption, it would be a wonderful thing if a couple experienced with diabetes could find it in their hearts to adopt a diabetic baby or older child.

(NOTE: a very useful book, *The Baby Team; A Positive Approach to Pregnancy with Diabetes*, is available for $2.50 from Monoject Division of Sherwood Medical, Department T.I., 1831 Olive Street, St. Louis, Missouri 63103. Its only flaw is that it doesn't discuss home blood sugar testing in conjunction with pregnancy.)

What is the best contraceptive for a diabetic woman to use?

Two British physicians, J. M. Steel and L. J. P. Duncan, studied the use of contraceptives by insulin-dependent diabetic women. Their conclusions reported in the November–December, 1980 issue of *Diabetes Forecast*, were:

The pill. They warn against the use of the combined pill, which contains both estrogen and progestogen. Women who use this pill have a higher incidence of heart attacks and strokes. If used at all by diabetic women, it should be only for the shortest possible time. They recommend instead the progestogen only pill.

The IUD. They consider this to be unacceptable for diabetic women because it is highly ineffective. (It has also been known to cause infections.)

The diaphragm. This, along with the progestogen-only pill, is on their "best choice" list. The failure rate for mechanical devices like this and the condom is, they say, due mainly to using them incorrectly or "forgetting" to use them.

Sterilization. For women who are certain they don't want to become pregnant in the future, sterilization (obviously!) is the most reliable method.

One diabetic woman we talked to said she thinks the safest and most reliable method of contraception is a husband with a vasectomy.

And, finally, our editor, who feels we should present every possible option in this book, offers the reminder, "There's always celibacy."

How do I cut the high cost of being a diabetic?

You're right to worry about costs. Being a diabetic can be an expensive proposition and the expenses rise every year with inflation and new discoveries in diabetes care.

The number one way to keep costs down is to practice preventive maintenance, just as you do with a car. If you keep your diabetes in control and keep yourself healthy, you'll keep yourself out of the hospital. Hospitalization is the most horrendous expense of all.

If you have a choice of health insurance plans where you work, be sure to investigate them to see which one pays for the most diabetes expenses. Some now pay for blood sugar testing materials and meters and some even reimburse you for insulin and syringes.

Often insurance companies initially refuse to pay for something like Chemstrips or Dextrometers and Dextrostix but if you keep haranguing them and submitting letters from your doctor (or lawyer!) and evidence of other plans that pay, they sometimes will eventually (and reluctantly) come around. It's worth the fight, because not only will you save money yourself, but you'll make it easier for diabetics who come after you to get reimbursement for their basic needs.

When you're working on health insurance claims, be sure to keep pointing out to them how much money they'll save in the long run if they pay for, say, home blood sugar testing materials, and you use them to keep yourself well and out of the hospital.

Incidentally, we've heard from health professionals that the best time to ask insurance companies to pay for home blood sugar testing equipment and supplies is right after a patient has been hospitalized with some diabetes problem. While the high hospital bills are fresh in its computerized memory, the insurance company is much more likely to pay for those things that will keep a diabetic healthy and out of the hospital. Of course, this is the hard way of getting the insurance companies to cough up and is hardly recommended.

When it comes to buying diabetes supplies, do a lot of comparison shopping. Prices vary tremendously from pharmacy to pharmacy. Sometimes you can even bargain with them for a discount if you buy in quantity.

Watch for sales on such things as Tes-Tape and disposable syringes and stock up. Watch for discount coupon offers from the manufacturers. You sometimes find these in *Diabetes Forecast* or at diabetes association meetings. Talk to other diabetics and see how they find ways of cutting costs.

Often you can save money by mail order. The American Association of Retired Persons pharmacies have very competitive prices on insulin, urine testing materials, and disposable syringes. You can join the association if you're fifty-five years old or older for a cost of $4.00 a year. (Write to the American

Association of Retired Persons, Membership Processing Department, P. O. Box 199, Long Beach, California 90801.) If you're too young, we can't see anything wrong with having an older relative join and order your supplies for you.

In *Diabetes Forecast*, mail-order "discount pharmacies" surface from time to time. Some of these require that you pay an annual membership fee of $12–$24, so you have to make sure you'll be ordering enough each year to make the investment worthwhile. Others may offer a special super-low price good for one order only. This is a way of getting you on their mailing list, but if you don't mind being on another mailing list, you do save a lot on the one order—and in spending for diabetes supplies, every penny counts.

We started the Sugarfree Center to try both to keep prices down and to discover and make available new products that improve diabetes care. (We test all of these out on June, our resident guinea pig.) We publish a bulletin that describes the products and includes any thrift tips we discover (see Reference Section: Directory of Services for Diabetics).

If you really put your mind to it, you can come up with a lot of ways to cut down on the costs of diabetes. For example, many people use their disposable syringes and needles several times until they grow too dull to be comfortable. (One fellow who dropped by the Sugarfree Center told us he used his fifteen or twenty times! In fact, he said he liked them better when they weren't so sharp!) After using the needle you should carefully recap it, very carefully because you don't want to hit the needle with the plastic cap and further dull it or bend it. Then place it in the refrigerator until the next use. (This prevents the growth of bacteria in case some got on it.)

When it comes to home blood sugar testing—an admittedly expensive proposition—there are many ways to save. Using Chemstrips bG or Dextrostix alone rather than buying a meter is, of course, a big saving, but if you need the accuracy of a meter, sometimes you can buy a used model secondhand (see Something for Everyone: How Can I Tell If My Diabetes Is in Control?).

With the Autolet you can cut costs a good bit over the years by ignoring the printed instructions that tell you to throw away the lancet and platform after each use. You can, in fact, keep using the same lancet until it gets dull. June usually uses hers around five times.

As for the platform, there is no need to ever change it unless it gets bent or broken. June has been using the same one for over two years. The ten platforms that come with the Autolet will probably be enough to last you through your next four or five incarnations.

While using the Autolet is admittedly the easiest and most painless way to get a blood sample for the test, you don't have to have one to do home blood sugar testing. You can prick your finger with a lancet or—even more of a saving—with an old insulin needle. This is how June did it in her early days of home blood sugar testing.

Now here's the Really Big Saving. We heard the rumor that some clever rascals were cutting their Chemstrip bG testing strips in half (lengthwise, of course) and thereby getting two tests for the price of one. This sounded like a great idea but we were afraid that cutting them might break some sort of seal and make the test inaccurate, so we conducted a little experiment. We took two Chemstrips bG from the same vial, cut one in half and left the other one whole. We then put a drop of 130 glucose testing solution on each and followed the standard procedure. At the end of the test they looked identical and the half strip was just as easy to read as the whole one.

Since we feared the cut might make the color unstable and cause it to fade out, we set the strips aside and checked them every week. Now it's three months later and the two strips still look identical. Needless to say, June has cut all her

Chemstrips bG in half. Additional benefit: It takes a smaller drop of blood to make the test with a half strip.

Unfortunately, if you're using a machine, you can't cut your testing stick in half.

Another way for a diabetic to save money—and to be healthier as well—is to stop using a lot of expensive processed foods. Cook from scratch whenever time allows. You eliminate all kinds of chemical nasties and overgenerous sugaring and salting, and you gain more vitamins and minerals when you use fresh vegetables and fruits and bake your own bread products from whole grains.

Now, from the foregoing, you can see that we have the utmost empathy for people who have trouble paying for their diabetes necessities and we try to figure out ways to cut costs. There are people, however, who have plenty of money yet who clamp their wallets and purses shut when it comes to spending for supplies that will help improve their health.

At the Sugarfree Center we've had people drive up in Cadillacs and Lincoln Continentals who would sit and orate about their annual Caribbean cruises and European tours, and their winter homes in Palm Springs, and their summer hideaways at the beach, and then anguish over their doctor requiring them to buy "all this expensive stuff" (an Autolet and Chemstrips bG totaling out at around $40.00). They would mutter that they hoped they wouldn't have to "keep spending all this money" on testing their blood sugar for very long. Some would even decide to go home and think about it before springing for the supplies.

As Diane Victor, the Diabetes Teaching Nurse at Valley Presbyterian Hospital in Van Nuys, California, says, "Some diabetics have to get their priorities in order."

Ron Brown, the young diabetic who works with us, agrees, "You can't enjoy any of your other activities if you don't take care of your health." Since he's a normal human being, Ron would certainly prefer not to have diabetes and to buy a one-day ski lift ticket at Mammoth Mountain (currently $17) rather than a bottle of Chemstrips bG (currently under $17), or take his girl friend out to dinner (in all probability a $25 jaunt these days) rather than buy an Autolet for the same price. But he has his priorities—and his testing materials—and his health.

Will I be able to get insurance as a diabetic?

That depends on the kind of insurance you're interested in getting.

Automobile insurance. According to Henry Helfman, a North Hollywood insurance agent (and a diabetic), there should be no trouble if you're in good control. (Here's yet another reason to take good care of yourself.) If they ask on the form if you're a diabetic, naturally you have to tell them. In that case, they'll probably ask you to produce a letter from your doctor saying that your diabetes is in control.

If they don't ask, we don't see any point in saying, "Hey there, Insurance Company, I'm a diabetic. Don't you want to hassle me?" Personal experience: June's automobile insurance company has never asked; she has never told.

Life insurance. Mr. Helfman tells us that if you're under control (again with evidence required) and you take less than forty units of insulin—or don't take insulin at all—you should have no more difficulty getting life insurance than a nondiabetic.

Of special interest is a new program from the Security-Connecticut Life Insurance Company for children with diabetes. Diabetic children ages six and up can be insured *without a physical examination,* and they will be able to continue their policies at guaranteed rates up to the age of thirty-seven regardless of any changes in their health. (For information, write to Security-Connecticut Life Insurance Company, Security Drive, Avon, Connecticut 06001.)

Health Insurance. If you or your spouse or, if you're a minor, your parents work for a company or government agency with a group plan, you'll be taken care of, diabetic or not. If you have to take out an individual policy, then as a study reported in *Diabetes in the News* put it, "Your chances . . . are mighty slim." In all likelihood, you may not be able to get a policy or they may try to exclude coverage for all diabetes-related problems. In that case, the policy would be next to worthless, because insurance companies, being how they are, would probably find a way to relate anything that goes wrong with you to diabetes.

But don't feel you're being picked on because you're a diabetic. As Mr. Helfman explained to us, individual health insurance policies are a pretty rotten deal for everybody, with high prices and exclusions galore. It's all part of the trend in modern society for groups to get favored treatment in everything from air travel to Chinese dinners.

So get with a group if you possibly can. In the library where we work, there are women who have taken clerical jobs mainly to get the excellent health benefits for themselves and their families. In a sense that's not a bad idea. If you have a choice between two jobs and everything else is equal, select the one with the better health plan.

To find out the latest developments in the field of insurance for diabetics, write the American Diabetes Association (see Reference Section: Directory of Services for Diabetics). They evaluate all new plans and make them known to members, and there *are* new plans coming out all the time. Fortunately, insurance for diabetics is not the problem that it used to be. Now you only have the problems with insurance that nondiabetics have, and those are problems enough for anybody.

Will diabetes keep me from getting a job?

It didn't keep actress Mary Tyler Moore, radio and TV personality Gary Owens, hockey star Bobby Clarke, prominent physician Peter Forsham or McDonald's restaurant tycoon Ray Krock from getting the jobs they wanted. Why would it keep you from any career you choose? The truth is that the great majority of diabetics have the same employment opportunities and limitations as nondiabetics. So if you're qualified for a particular position, go after it positively and aggressively. Be up front about your diabetes. If the subject comes up with an employer, point out that diabetes develops a sane lifestyle and great self-discipline. These in turn lead to a superior performance on the job.

For the one million or so diabetics who take insulin, we do have to report on a few negatives. You should avoid jobs where you could endanger yourself or others during insulin reactions. It wouldn't be wise for you to seek jobs with high-speed machinery or climbing telephone poles, for example. Legally, there are certain restrictions, too. The federal government does not allow diabetics on insulin to enter the armed forces, to pilot airplanes, or to drive trucks or buses in interstate commerce. Also, it's inadvisable to aim for certain jobs with long and irregular working hours combined with potential emergency situations like police officer, firefighter, or airline flight attendants.

If you should run into job discrimination because of diabetes, don't hesitate to fight it. Federal regulations have made it illegal for most major employers to reject you solely because you have diabetes. You can file a complaint if you run into this situation. The law which protects you is Title V of the Rehabilitation Act passed by Congress in 1973. For details on how to file, write the American Diabetes Association for a copy of "Employment Opportunities and Protections for Diabetics."

Before this law came into effect, diabetics sometimes did have to resort to extremes to get jobs. A friend of ours told us that her husband, who has diabetes, desperately needed a job when they were first married and he had just graduated from college as a chemical engineer. She was pregnant. They had no money. Jobs were in short supply and he couldn't afford to take chances losing an opportunity because of diabetes. He heard of an opening with an engineering firm. He knew this firm required a physical before hiring. So he smuggled a little vial of his wife's urine into the examination with him. When he was asked to provide a specimen, he provided hers.

When he came home, his wife asked him how his scheme had worked. "Great," he said, "they didn't suspect a thing." Then his face clouded. "Say," he said, "what if they run some kind of test on that urine and it shows that I'm pregnant?"

They didn't and he got the job.

One admonition. We talked to the head of the handicapped program on the college campus where we work. He said that after he had fought reluctant employers, citing Title V, and finally managed to get certain of his students jobs, they would work for a short period of time and then try to get a semiphony disability retirement based on the very health problem he had claimed wouldn't affect their performance. This calls the whole program into question and makes it hard if not impossible for others with similar health problems to get jobs later on—to say nothing about how it shreds the moral fiber of the person crying disabled wolf.

Can I drink alcohol? _____

Here you have one of the great diabetes controversies. Many doctors say absolutely no to alcohol. Not a drop. Others say it's all right in moderation. June has a joke which has a grain of truth in it. Question: "What did you do when your doctor said you couldn't drink?" Answer: "I changed doctors." There is some validity in changing doctors, if you insist on drinking and he or she insists that you don't. There is no point in going to a doctor if you intend to defy instructions, or, even worse, sneak off and do something forbidden.

Actually, an excellent case can be made for a diabetic not to drink at all. Even alcoholic beverages that don't contain carbohydrate, such as gin, vodka, bourbon, scotch, and dry wines, do contain calories. If you have a weight problem, the additional calories of the drink will augment this problem. If you say, "OK, I'll figure the calories of the drink in my diet and cut out something else," then that something else you cut out will have food value that alcohol lacks and your body will be deprived of the nutrition it needs.

Then, too, drinking can get you in deep trouble, especially if you're on insulin. Let's take a hypothetical situation. It's the end of the day. Work is over. You're tired. You decide you'll have a pick-me-up drink before going home. You do. Then maybe you have another. Your judgment is suspended and your mind is a little fuzzy. You forget it's time for you to eat. In fact, it's past time. The alcohol unaccompanied by food further lowers your blood sugar and it also impairs the liver's ability to release emergency glucose.

You leave the bar and start walking several blocks to where your car is parked. Hypoglycemia comes over you. You stagger, stumble, and finally fall. You lose consciousness. Somebody calls the police to come pick up the drunk. The police arrive and, smelling alcohol on your breath, haul you off to the drunk tank to sober up Very bad trouble.

Besides the dire possibilities of this scenario, there is the additional possibility that the alcohol may throw off your medication or alter the effect of your insulin. Oral drugs combined with alcohol sometimes cause nausea, sweating and dizziness. And an out-of-control diabetic shouldn't drink a drop.

Heavy drinking can result in long-range problems for a diabetic. The March–April 1980 issue of *Diabetes Care* reported a study by David McCullogh and others of over 500 diabetic men. The heavy drinkers in the group had a much higher incidence of painful diabetic neuropathy than the others did.

Isn't there anything to say in favor of drinking for diabetics?

The case *for* drinking is weaker than the one against it, but it is still there. For many people a glass of wine is a pleasurable adjunct to a meal. It is, in fact, for some national groups as much a part of the meal as the food. A small amount of alcohol is relaxing, and on festive occasions it makes you feel a part of the celebration. It would, for example, be sad not to have a glass of champagne at your own wedding. One glass of wine or a single mild drink makes you feel not nearly so left out and deprived as total abstention does.

Even with your doctor's approval, however, before having a glass of anything, you should do a little self-analysis of your drinking habits. Do you drink for the taste or for the effect? Are you the kind of person who can stop with one mild drink or one glass of wine? Or are you the kind who, once the first drink is down so are the barriers, and you have another, then another? If so, then don't take the first sip. There is no more lethal combination than diabetes and alcoholism.

Early on, we developed a philosophy about diabetic drinking, and with fourteen years of experience behind us, it still holds. There are two reasons for a diabetic *not* to drink: The first is if alcohol means nothing to you and the second is if alcohol means everything to you.

If I decide to drink, which drinks and how much of them can I have?

You have to learn which drinks contain sugar, which are high in carbohydrates, and how many calories they all contain.

Whatever you drink has to be figured into your meal plan and the calories counted. Alcoholic drinks are usually calculated as fat exchanges, although you can also substitute them for bread exchanges. Naturally, you can't mix liquor with orange juice or tomato juice without counting those exchanges also. And you have to avoid such mixers as ginger ale, tonic, and other sweetened soft drinks.

The alcoholic drinks that don't contain sugar or carbohydrates are dry white wines (including champagne), dry red and rosé wines, white vermouth, whiskey, gin, vodka, scotch, rum, brandy, and tequila. A four-ounce glass of wine is about 80 calories; a four-ounce glass of vermouth is about 140 calories. The hard liquors are calculated according to their proof. The higher the proof, the more calories. As an example, 86-proof alcohol is 71 calories an ounce; 100-proof alcohol is 83 calories an ounce. Beer is 156 calories per twelve-ounce bottle, but it also contains about the same amount of carbohydrate as a bread exchange (13 grams). Light beer is only 96 calories on the average and contains the equivalent of ½ bread exchange in carbohydrate. Liqueurs and cordials have to be avoided entirely as they contain sugar—sometimes as much as 50 percent sugar. Appetizer and dessert wines, like sweet sherry, port, and muscatel, are also too sweet for diabetics. (*The Diabetic's Total Health Book* contains a complete list of alcoholic beverages with their carbohydrates and caloric values.)

The general recommendation is to limit alcoholic beverages to 6 percent of your daily caloric allotment. For instance, if you're on a 1,500-calorie-a-day diet, you could have one four-ounce glass of wine (80 calories) or one generous ounce of 86-proof liquor (71 calories) in soda or a sugarfree mixer. You could also have it in orange juice, if you counted that as one of your fruit exchanges. If you are on a 3,000-calorie-a-day diet, you could drink twice that much (but you wouldn't *have* to, of course).

Can *diabetics travel?* _____

Not only *can* but *should.*

If you need to travel for your job, there's no reason to let diabetes stop you. As a matter of fact, because of your good health habits, you may well be more bright and alert and ready for the work than the other business people who may feel a little headachy from the airline cocktails or drowsy from carousing.

But even more important is the travel you should do for pleasure and mind-expansion. To our way of thinking, the vacation spent puttering around the house is not a vacation at all. A true vacation gets you away from home and away from the routine demands on your time and the routine worries that constantly nibble on your subconscious.

The strange thing is that if you just get away for a short time—even a weekend—you feel so restored that it's as if you've had a month-long holiday.

If you're nervous about handling your diabetes away from home, you might try our expanding circle method of travel. Make your first trip a weekend jaunt to a very nearby town or, if you live in a large city, to another part of the same city. You can pretend you're on the opposite side of the earth, but you know you can get home fast or get in touch with your doctor, if there's an emergency. (There never is.)

When you've proved to yourself that staying in a hotel and eating all of your meals out poses no problems to you or your diabetes, expand the circle farther by going some place about 500 miles away. Next travel all the way across the country to a place you've always wanted to visit. Then try Canada or Hawaii—both seem foreign and yet they pose no language or food problems.

Finally, if the current state of the dollar and your own bank account allow, go to Europe or Asia or Australia or Africa or even Antarctica, if that's your strange pleasure. For the truth is that a diabetic can travel anywhere that diabetics live and of course, that's every country on earth.

Now that you're all hyped up and ready to go, here are a few of our favorite travel tips and precautions.

1. Take double quantities of all diabetes and other medical supplies that you use. It may not be easy to find them, especially overseas, and besides, who wants to spend vacation time shopping in pharmacies? If you're a belt and suspenders type, as June is, carry half your supplies in one place and half in another so if you should lose a purse or piece of luggage, you'll still be covered.

2. Try to go to just one place. In the U.S. make it one city or national park or resort area; overseas just one country. (A few years ago we actually went just to Rome for three weeks.) If you don't try to gulp down the whole world on a single vacation, you'll spend more time being there rather than going to a lot of different theres. You'll have more time on your feet exploring or playing than on your seat in a car or bus or train or plane. Your diabetes will show its appreciation.

In foreign travel, if you go to only one country, you'll be able to do research ahead of time into the cuisine to make your meals easier to figure, and more fun as well. You'll also be able to learn a few appropriate phrases in the language. ("I am a diabetic." "Where is the rest room?" "Quick! Get me some orange juice!")

3. Sports vacations are wonderful. Not only do you get healthful and restoring exercise while you're there but you can also take lessons to acquire (or hone) a skill like tennis or golf or skiing that will enrich and enhealth your whole life.

4. Two short vacations are better than one long one. You get the welcome release of a holiday at two different times of the year instead of just one. And it's true that it becomes weary-making to stay away from home for too long. June prefers vacations of one or two weeks, but if she's going overseas,

she's willing to stretch it to three. Her basic rule: "I come home when all my clothes are dirty."

5. Take along two pairs of broken-in (*not* broken-down) shoes. If possible, change your shoes in the middle of the day. This helps prevent blisters. Walk and walk and walk and walk. You'll see more and get to *eat* more that way.

6. As you start your trip, make it a point to slip into what Olympic Gold Medal marathon runner, and attorney, Frank Shorter calls his "travel mode." This means keeping relaxed and making a conscious effort not to let anything bother you. If there's a flight delay, no matter. If a crying baby is seated nearby, no matter. If someone whaps your ear with a flight bag when putting it in the overhead compartment, no matter. Remain in a semimeditative state, a kind of "serene mellowness," as Shorter puts it. Getting angry and upset over the inevitable annoyances associated with travel only hurts (and raises the blood sugar of) one person: you.

Another Shorter travel tip is to be especially pleasant to any of the service people you deal with on a trip. He finds the courtesy is usually returned in kind and often serves to iron out potential wrinkles in your trip (and on your brow).

Follow these rules and, indeed, the longest and most grueling of flights, or bus, train, or car trips will seem shorter.

7. Write for the following booklets and pamphlets:

a. *Vacationing With Diabetes, Not From Diabetes,* a free booklet from E. R. Squibb & Sons, Inc., Lawrenceville-Princeton Road, Princeton, New Jersey 08540.

b. A list of English-speaking doctors and hospitals all over the world from IAMAT, 350 Fifth Avenue, Suite 5620, New York, New York 10001. There's no fixed price for this. Just send a donation to keep them operating. Along with the list you receive twenty-four World Climate Charts with safety of water, milk, and food indicated and suggestions for clothing appropriate for the climate.

c. The names of diabetes specialists in the areas in which you'll be traveling. These can be supplied by the International Diabetes Federation (IDF) if you write to Mr. James G. L. Jackson, Executive Secretary, 10 Queen Anne Street, London W1M0BD, England.

d. *Holidays and Travel for Diabetics*, a helpful pamphlet available from the British Diabetic Association. [The address is the same as the IDF (above). Cost is 25 cents American money, 40 pence British money.]

8. Relax and have fun.

How can I get special diabetic meals on airlines?

You request them when you buy your tickets and the agent relays your order to the airline. If you change your flight number, you must inform the airline so that they can switch your meal order, too.

Which airlines offer special diet trays? Virtually all of the major foreign and domestic ones. Some have standard diabetic meals, while others ask that you specify exactly what you want and their catering service will prepare it for you.

The way the special meal service works is that you notify one of the flight attendants as you board the plane that they're carrying a special meal for you. If you don't identify yourself at the beginning of the flight, your chances of getting the meal are nil.

We've found, however, that the special diabetic meal is sometimes less appetizing and occasionally even less diabetically appropriate than the standard fare. Consequently we often just settle for the regular meal or bring our own food, because after all, a diabetic can eat very little when immobilized on an airplane anyway. It's better not to concentrate on food but rather on drinking lots of water (so you won't get dehydrated from the altitude) and walking up and down the aisle as often as you can to keep your circulation chugging along. Alcohol is not a good idea either, as it, too, is dehydrating. When it comes to diabetics on an airplane, getting there is generally not half the fun. Be sure to bring along a good book.

═══ SHORT SUBJECTS ═══

How come I didn't have any symptoms of diabetes when my case was diagnosed?

You were one of the thousands of hidden diabetics—people who have diabetes and don't realize it. You're one of the smart (or lucky) ones. You caught diabetes early by a urine or blood sugar test before it had done any real damage.

If you neglect your diabetes in the future, that's when you may begin to experience the classic symptoms of more advanced diabetes: excessive urination and thirst, increased appetite, rapid loss of weight, irritability, weakness and fatigue, and nausea and vomiting. These indicate ketoacidosis, which if untreated will lead to coma and ultimately to death. These are the symptoms that usually strike children and adolescents suddenly.

Most people who get diabetes between the ages of thirty-five and sixty have a different set of symptoms, though they may also have any of the above. Generally, the warning signals for this age group are drowsiness, itching, blurred vision, tingling and numbness in feet, easy fatigue, skin infections, and slow healing. People of this age group often have two additional clues that diabetes may be in the offing: they are overweight and they have a family history of diabetes.

Isn't there a kind of diabetes that has nothing to do with blood sugar? _____

Yes. It's called *diabetes insipidus* and it is a problem of the hypothalamus rather than the pancreas. The hypothalamus produces an antidiuretic hormone which limits the formation of urine in the kidneys. When something (tumor, infection, or injury) damages the hypothalamus, interfering with the production of the hormone, excessive urination (along with excessive water drinking) is the result.

Diabetes insipidus can also be hereditary and, like diabetes mellitus, can't be cured but can be controlled by the use of a hormone. Strangely enough, this hormone is sometimes taken in the form of a nasal spray. (Too bad insulin can't be snorted in this way!)

Diabetes insipidus is also called "water diabetes" to differentiate it from "sugar diabetes."

What does "borderline diabetes" mean? _____

It means nothing. As of 1979, the term is no longer used. In that year the National Diabetes Data Group came up with a new system for classifying diabetes and this classification was endorsed by the Board of Directors of the American Diabetes Association at their annual meeting.

The new classification system wiped out such fuzzy and often misunderstood terms as "borderline diabetes," "chemical diabetes," "subclinical diabetes," "asymptomatic diabetes," and "latent diabetes." All of these terms were replaced with "impaired glucose tolerance."

In a report in the December, 1979 issue of *Diabetes*, it was pointed out that impaired glucose tolerance is not diabetes and the use of the label "diabetes" for people with "marginal" blood levels, "can invoke social, psychological, and economic sanctions that are unjustified in the light of the lack of severity of their glucose intolerance." (Translation: These people shouldn't be denied jobs that are forbidden to diabetics.)

This glucose tolerance test graph (Figure 4, page 116) shows the difference in glucose levels among a nondiabetic, a person with impaired glucose tolerance, and a diabetic.

As the March–April 1980 *Diabetes Forecast* points out, "While some people whose blood-glucose levels are somewhat elevated *do* develop diabetes, many people subsequently have normal tests and continue to test 'normal' indefinitely."

Our personal opinion is that if you have impaired glucose tolerance you should follow the diabetic lifestyle just to be on the safe side. But then we feel that *everybody* should follow the diabetic lifestyle.

What do they mean when they say you have Type I or Type II diabetes?

Type I is another and newer term for juvenile or insulin-dependent diabetes. This kind of diabetes usually occurs in children, but it can occur at any age. That's why it's a preferred term over juvenile diabetes. It now covers people like June, who got it as an adult but has to take insulin.

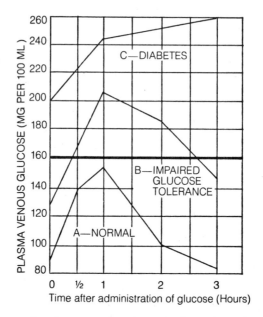

FIGURE 4 The three people represented on this graph each had 100 grams of glucose administered by mouth. One person (A-Normal) is nondiabetic. One person (B-Normal) has impaired glucose tolerance. And the other person (C-DM) is diabetic, either insulin-dependent or non-insulin-dependent. You can see that the nondiabetic's body has removed most of the glucose from circulation within two hours. In the diabetic, whose glucose levels were already too high, the glucose level shot even higher than at first, and three hours later, the levels had not yet begun to drop. The person with impaired glucose tolerance has a curve similar to that of the nondiabetic, except that it is somewhat higher. Also, at the end of two hours, this person's glucose level had dropped only slightly, whereas the nondiabetic's blood-glucose level had returned to normal.

Courtesy of Gerald R. Cooper, M.D., Ph.D., Diabetes Forecast, March–April 1980, p. 39. Copyright 1980 by the American Diabetes Association. Reprinted from Diabetes Forecast with permission.

Type II is the newer term for adult-onset, non-insulin-dependent diabetes.

Types I and II can be further broken down into types Ia

and Ib to distinguish between those who produce no insulin of their own and those (again, like June) who produce some but not enough. Type II can be broken down into IIa and IIb, with the former referring to the overweight (or as the medical profession prefers, obese) and the latter to the nonobese.

Does getting emotionally upset affect my diabetes?

An emotional upset has about the same effect on blood sugar as chocolate chip cookies. A fight with an intimate, a boost in rent, a week of final examinations, any stressful event in your life can send diabetes dramatically out of control. The strange thing is that even if something favorable takes place in your life, that, too, can raise blood sugar. When we were consultants on a tour to Hawaii for diabetics, several of the participants told us they got out of control with the excitement of packing for the trip.

We are so convinced of the need for diabetics to learn how to handle the stresses of contemporary life that we wrote an entire book on the theme. *The Diabetic's Total Health Book* explains why tensions and stresses have a negative effect on diabetes, what stressors you can avoid, and how to develop techniques to keep those you can't avoid from upsetting your control. A good portion of that book is devoted to instruction in relaxation therapies. These therapies—exercise, self-hypnosis, biofeedback, meditation, and guided imagery—are the best preventive medicine ever invented. Each of you should start practicing the ones that appeal to you most. You'll particularly enjoy practicing our unique all-purpose relaxers: laughter and hugs, both of which will enhance your life and the lives of all those around you.

The Diabetic's Total Health Book is available in hardback from J. P. Tarcher, Inc., and in paperback from Pocket Books. If you can't find it in your bookstore, write to us at the Sugarfree Center.

How much should I weigh? _____

A very simple and convenient test of the correctness of your weight is to pinch up your flesh just below your ribs at your waistline. Pressing the flesh between your thumb and fore-finger, you should find a thickness of between one-half and one inch. If the pinch test reveals more flesh than that, you're too fat.

Another guideline is to think back and recall what you weighed in your early twenties. That's when most of us are at our ideal weight (assuming you weren't overweight *then*). Tables 2 and 3 will help you find your ideal weight, as they show what is considered both slender and normal for college students. Find your height on the men's or women's chart and you'll have a target weight for slender or normal for yourself.

TABLE 2
IDEAL WEIGHTS FOR YOUNG MEN

Height (in.)	Slender (lbs.)	Normal (lbs.)
63	121	131
64	124	134
65	128	138
66	131	141
67	134	145
68	138	149
69	141	152
70	145	156
71	148	160
72	152	165
73	156	169
74	160	173
75	164	178
76	168	182
77	173	187
78	177	192

TABLE 3
IDEAL WEIGHTS FOR YOUNG WOMEN

Height (in.)	Slender (lbs.)	Normal (lbs.)
58	95	103
59	98	106
60	101	109
61	104	112
62	106	115
63	109	118
64	112	122
65	116	125
66	119	128
67	122	132
68	126	136
69	129	140
70	133	143
71	136	147
72	140	152
73	144	156
74	148	160

(The slender figure is preferable for diabetics, since that would lessen the demands on your pancreas.)

Incidentally, we don't favor the Metropolitan Life Insurance weight charts, because they tell average weights for Americans, and average in this country is not ideal. It's too heavy, especially for diabetics. Their charts are even revised periodically and the averages go up as Americans continue to eat too much for their sedentary lifestyle.

How can I make myself follow the diabetes diet?

You can conjure up horror stories in your imagination about the terrible things that will happen to you if you don't. But a strong positive approach is better. Make your meals so delicious and interesting that you *want* to follow your diet. Make your eating not a grim therapy, but a pleasurable delight. There are lots of gourmet cookbooks available for diabetics now (see Suggested Reading). Try new recipes. Try variations on old recipes. Try different herbs and spices. (Most of these are free, diabetically speaking.) And don't overlook the aesthetics of food serving. A few flowers on the table give you no extra carbohydrates or calories and do a lot toward making mealtime a pleasure.

This all holds especially true if you live alone. June, in her prediabetic days, often used to have for dinner what we called an "avocado sandwich maybe"; since whenever someone asked her what she was having for dinner, she usually responded vaguely, "Oh, I guess I'll have an avocado sandwich maybe," which meant she had no idea what she was going to have and didn't intend to make any plans. She was going to grab whatever she found in the refrigerator, if anything.

Now, June always has a well-planned and delicious meal that she eagerly looks forward to. Her appetite is also better. And strangely enough, although she's eating fewer calories, she's eating more—and more satisfying—food. This is because she's cut down on high calorie fats and cut out entirely high (and empty) calorie junk foods.

The most ghastly diabetic diet idea we've ever heard of is the result of a man's decision that calculating the diabetic diet is too much of a chore. He resolved to eat the same breakfast, the same lunch, and the same dinner every day. Ugh! Besides being lethally boring, this is nutritionally unsound. Diabetics need a lot of variety in their diets in order to make certain they're covering all the nutritional waterfronts. Not only that, but, as a home economist told us wryly, "You should eat a great variety of foods, because there are so many chemicals in everything these days, it's the only way you can avoid getting a big buildup of one chemical that might cause harmful side effects."

Is there anything I can eat all I want of without counting it in my diet?

Yes, you can eat all the unsweetened rhubarb, unsweetened cranberries, and unflavored gelatin that you can possibly hold.

But seriously, folks, you can hype up the flavors of your meals with herbs and spices without counting them. And you can eat as much of the following vegetables as you want, if you eat them raw: chicory; Chinese cabbage; endive; escarole; iceberg, butter, red leaf, or romaine lettuce; parsley; radishes; and watercress.

What things should I eat a lot of?

Well, you shouldn't eat a gigantic lot of anything. One of the basic principles of the diabetic diet is great variety but small quantity. You could, however, say that, compared to the average American's diet, a diabetic should eat a lot of fruits and vegetables, especially the latter.

Can I save up food exchanges from one meal and use them for the next?

Definitely not. One of the most important principles of the diabetic eating plan is having every meal well balanced and eating neither more nor less than is called for. A diabetic, especially an insulin-dependent one, would really get into trouble following the great American eating pattern of nothing much for breakfast, a light lunch, and a gorging session at night. As a matter of fact, all those nondiabetics who do follow this scheme are getting themselves into trouble, too. They don't feel their best, they don't function well, and they're putting on wads of fat.

The only exchange you can ever save up is your fat exchange. We don't mean that you can save fat exchanges for several days and then lap up a pint of whipping cream. It's more like saving one fat exchange from breakfast and one from lunch and using them at dinner. Even this shouldn't be a standard method of operating, only an occasional indulgence, and especially not when an increase in activity is planned after a particular meal.

Can a diabetic follow a vegetarian diet?

Of course. We consider the vegetarian diet extremely healthy for everyone and especially good for non-insulin-dependent diabetics who are overweight. In fact, Dr. Anderson's HCF Diet (see Something for Everyone: What Is the Diabetic Diet?) is as close as it can get to a vegetarian diet without being one.

Any diabetic who is (or wants to be) a vegetarian should get a copy of the Exchange List Supplements of Vegetarian Cookery published by the Washington, D.C. Area Affiliate of the ADA. It can be ordered for forty-five cents directly from the American Diabetes Association, Washington, D.C. Area Affiliate Inc., 7961 Eastern Avenue, Silver Spring, Maryland 20910. It is also included in the Appendix of *The Diabetic's Total Health Book* (see Reference Section: Suggested Reading).

Our all-time favorite vegetarian cookbook is *Laurel's Kitchen*, but there are several other excellent ones (see Reference Section: Suggested Reading).

The one problem we've heard about with a vegetarian diet is that it can be deficient in vitamin B$_{12}$, which can be taken in pill form but is much more effective when injected.

If you're an insulin taker and familiar with the injection process, you might ask your doctor about shooting your own B$_{12}$ as Barbara did (see For Concerned Family Members and Friends: How Do I Help the Diabetic in My Life?), and as a matter of fact still does, since we both are, like those who follow Dr. Anderson's diet, as close as we can get to a vegetarian without being one.

What about health foods for diabetics?

If you mean granola, home-baked bread, yogurt, soybeans, sunflower seeds, wheat germ, alfalfa sprouts, and all that, great! The more different foods you eat, the better. Just make certain that you know the calorie, protein, fat, and carbohydrate content (or exchange equivalent) of whatever you eat and limit your portions so that you stay within your diet.

June adores many health foods but finds she has to select them carefully, because many of these foods are laced with concentrated sweets—honey, coconut, dried fruits, brown sugar—and many of them are overpotent in fat, and calories. For instance, one-half cup of sunflower seeds is 280 calories and 26 grams of fat.

Most health breads are also heavier than ordinary bread. One slice will often equal almost two bread exchanges instead of one. You can check this out by weighing a slice. Bread is usually 50 percent carbohydrate, so a slice weighing sixty grams contains thirty grams of carbohydrate, or two bread exchanges.

A couple of words of warning about buying health foods. They tend to be terribly overpriced, and sometimes, rumor has it, those costly, organically grown fruits and vegetables aren't grown in any special way at all.

Why is it that I can eat a meal and not show any sugar afterwards and then eat the very same meal again and spill sugar?

This frustrating phenomenon happens to most diabetics. We've read that it can be explained by changes in the body's metabolism from day to day or, indeed, from hour to hour. Also, it stands to reason that variations in the amount of daily exercise, variations in the measurements of insulin and the absorption at different injection sites, as well as one's emotional state would influence what any specific meal does to the blood sugar.

That's why it's so important for you to monitor your own blood sugar so you can know when these strange things are happening and make the necessary adjustments.

Do I have to measure my food?

Yes, it's the only way to be sure you're getting the amount of food your diet specifies. It's not easy to recognize a half cup of orange juice or rice, unless you've measured them out a few times, and six grams of beef would be even harder. A food scale is a good investment in the beginning of your diabetic days to get you on the right measuring track.

If you're really conscientious about weighing and measuring your food at first, you'll be amazed at how quickly you learn to eye-measure or, as with bread, hand-weigh, when you're out to dinner at a friend's house or in a restaurant. (Hint: sometimes it helps to discreetly nudge your food into little piles, the better to estimate the quantity.) You may get so good at this eye-measuring and hand-weighing that you can do weight- and quantity-guessing parlor tricks, like the guy who guesses weights at the circus. Of course, the real and worthwhile trick is using your skill to eat the exact amount of food on your diet.

Is fructose a good sweetener for a diabetic?

Fructose is being promoted now because it is sweeter than table sugar and you can use less of it for the same amount of sweet taste. Therefore, you get fewer calories. Also, the body handles it in such a way that it does not cause the quick and high elevations of blood sugar that regular sugar does. This is why it is claimed to be especially useful for diabetics. Furthermore, it does not require insulin for use by the body.

Sounds great, doesn't it?

Wouldn't you know there's always a catch. Nobody has yet figured out how increasing the amount of fructose in your diet (it occurs naturally in fruits) affects you in the long run. And if you do use it, you can't just "ingest it freely" as dietitians like to put it. You have to count each tablespoon as one of your fruit exchanges. And don't forget that although fructose doesn't need insulin at the start of the digestion process, after it's been stored in the liver it requires insulin when it's released again as glucose.

Therefore, again we are up in the air. The American Diabetes Association says there is not enough evidence to either accept or reject the use of fructose by diabetics. It almost presents enough of a quandary to make you give up sweets altogether.

Are artificial sweeteners all right for a diabetic? _____

Well, they're better than downing an equal quantity of sugar. An occasional artificially sweetened drink is pleasant. We've found an especially good artificially sweetened tonic called Thintonic. Certain desserts like custard, gelatin, and pudding would be pretty dismal without some sweetening, and, if the sweetening is artificial, you can eat a more normal-size portion than if you were using sugar. June also confesses a fondness for Alba Fit'N Frosty milk shakes and their hot chocolate, both of which are artificially sweetened.

It's not, however, a good idea to load up on huge quantities of anything, especially anything chemical. You never know when it's going to dawn on the Food and Drug Administration that some chemical on their GRAS (generally recognized as safe) list has harmful side effects, as happened with cyclamates and as could happen with saccharine. One way to avoid getting too much of any one chemical is to buy several different brands of artificial sweeteners and alternate using them.

Much better than trying to fake a sweet taste with chemicals, however, is to lose your taste for sweets. If you're a sweet freak, this probably strikes you as utterly impossible. But the plain truth is that if you stop eating concentrated sweets, you eventually come to dislike them. Then it is an affront to you if someone disguises the beautiful, natural flavor of a plate of strawberries by heaping it with sugar or several squirts of the artificial stuff.

Another good reason for not relying heavily on artificial sweeteners is that they help you, in effect, deny that you have diabetes. As we say again and again, acceptance is one of the most important factors in leading a successful and happy diabetic life.

Why am I supposed to read the label on all food products I buy? Aren't all brands more or less alike?

Brands are not only *not* alike, they are very different. Only by reading the fine print on the label can you know, for instance, whether a certain can of grapefruit juice contains sugar or not. Some brands do and some don't, and it's important for you to choose a brand that is unsweetened.

It's amazing how many food products have sugar thrown in. Fruits in heavy syrup are typical. You have to really search to find the few fruits, frozen or canned, that are unsweetened. Cans of vegetables often contain sugar, as do canned meats, bottled salad dressings, frozen dinners, and endless other convenience foods. Even *salt* contains sugar—read the label if you doubt us.

Since the ban on cyclamates, there's even been a confusion with diet soft drinks. You have to realize that the term *artificially sweetened* does not necessarily mean without sugar. Drinks sweetened with saccharin often contain some sugar to counteract saccharin's bitter taste. On lo-cal drinks watch for the words *sugarless* and *sugarfree*. But even that's not a guarantee of safety. By law only sucrose counts as sugar so you'll have to watch for the many chemical terms used to specify different kinds of sugars: glucose, fructose, dextrose, sucrose maltose, lactose, dextrin, and sorbitol—just to name a few (see Reference Section: How Sweet It Is, for a complete list).

The nutrition label now required on food is also very helpful to diabetics. To refresh your memory, it tells the serving size, number of calories, grams of protein, carbohydrate, and fat. This information is important to you because it can help you measure your food and fit it into your diet.

Incidentally, ingredient lists on labels are arranged according to the weight of each ingredient in descending order. The heaviest is listed first; the lightest, last. The lightest ingredients are usually those unintelligible chemical additives for which the American food processors have become famous. If you're baffled by what's going to be going into your stomach—and who wouldn't be with the likes of sodium metasilicate, calcium hydroxide, BHT, etc.—we suggest you read one of the current books which explains why these chemicals are in the foods we buy and what they do to it and to us (see Reference Section: Suggested Reading).

Can I avoid all sugar?

It's not easy. In fact if you eat out or use processed foods, it's virtually impossible. Sugar sneaks in everywhere, and sometimes it jumps in with both feet. Just take a look at this list of "Hidden Sugar Traps," supplied to us by Boston diabetologist and Harvard Medical School professor, Dr. Stephen Podolsky.

HIDDEN SUGAR TRAPS
PERCENTAGE OF REFINED SUGAR IN
COMMERICAL FOOD PRODUCTS

Jell-O Cherry Gelatin Dessert	82.6%
Coffee-Mate Non-Dairy Creamer	65.4%
Cremora Non-Dairy Creamer	56.9%
Hershey's Milk Chocolate	51.4%
Shake 'N Bake Barbecue Style	50.9%
Sara Lee Chocolate Original Butter Recipe Cake	35.9%
Wish-Bone Russian Dressing	30.2%
Heinz Tomato Ketchup	28.9%

Quaker 100% Natural Cereal	23.9%
Hamburger Helper	23.0%
Sealtest Chocolate Ice Cream	21.4%
Birds Eye Cool Whip	21.0%
Libby's Sliced Peaches	17.9%
Wyler's Beef Bouillon Cubes	14.8%
Dannon Blueberry Low Fat Yogurt	13.7%
Ritz Crackers	11.8%
Del Monte Whole Kernel Corn	10.7%
Skippy Creamy Peanut Butter	9.2%
Coca Cola	8.8%
Ragu Spaghetti Sauce	6.2%

When you cook from scratch at home, you can do pretty well at avoiding sugar, although occasional grains of sugar are necessary for chemical reactions. For example, we used to worry over the fact that when you make your own bread you need some sugar to activate the yeast. We even tried (unsuccessfully) to use mashed apple instead.

Happily, though, a report by Dr. Jean Meyer in his newspaper column put our minds at ease on that subject, ". . . the sugar used is no longer in the finished loaf. It is broken down mainly to carbon dioxide, which causes the dough to expand, and ethyl alcohol, most of which is vaporized during baking." Of course this applies only to adding a small amount of sugar—one-two tablespoons per two-loaf batch—and not to throwing in the large quantities used in sweet breads.

All fruits contain a natural sugar that can't be avoided unless you avoid the fruit itself. The action of the sugar, however, is slowed down by the fibers in the fruit, so it doesn't jolt your system the way the juice alone does. That's why we advocate always eating the whole fruit and using juices only to counteract insulin reactions.

In Canada you may have even more trouble avoiding sugar. It was pointed out in the September–October 1980 issue of *Diabetes Forecast* that Canadian diet sodas such as Tab and Fresca contain some sugar because the use of cyclamates and saccharine is banned in manufactured foods. This is ironic because both artificial sweeteners are sold in markets and drugstores there. (American diabetics often toddle across the border to stock up on the cyclamates they can't buy at home.)

At any rate, Pat Steele of the Canadian Bureau of Nutritional Services advises diabetics to look for the label "sugar free" when buying soft drinks.

How can I eat the diabetic diet without imposing it on my family?

What have you got against your family? Don't you want them to be healthy? Do you want to be the only one who feels well and looks good? Shame on you. You should *insist* that they follow the diabetic diet and eat well-balanced meals that include fresh fruits and vegetables, more whole grains, and less sugar and fats. The diabetes diet is, after all, the perfect diet for everybody. We don't mean by this that everyone in the family will eat the same amount as the diabetic. If you have a strapping, seventeen-year-old, football player son, he's going to need a heap more of calories to carry him through the day than you do. But he should get his calories from the same kinds of food you're eating.

It's not as if you are torturing your family. Diabetic meals, when prepared with imagination, are as good or better than those that would throw you off your diet. When June has guests, she always serves them diabetic meals. After stowing away the artichoke vinaigrette, broiled salmon steak with horseradish, sherried carrots, homemade muffins, and fresh pineapple with mint, they look at her incredulously and say, "*That* was a diabetic meal? I could happily eat diabetic meals the rest of my life." They could and they should.

You see, the ill wind of diabetes does blow some good. It wafts the families of diabetics toward good eating habits. It may extend their lives as much as it extends the diabetics' lives. Barbara claims that June's diabetes is the best thing that ever happened to her, Barbara, in terms of decent nutrition. As she says, "If you really are what you eat, I used to be greasy doughnut. Now, thanks to you, I'm more like a crunchy apple."

What happens if I break my diet?

If you do it once, you'll probably do it again and again and again. And each time you do it and run your blood sugar up, you risk damage to the body and the development of the serious complications of diabetes—heart disease and stroke, blindness, kidney and nerve damage, and gangrene of the feet.

The classic rationalizations are "Once won't hurt," "I can get away with it," "It's Christmas," "I can't offend the hostess," "It's my birthday," and "I'll be conspicuous." Consider yourself in a worse predicament than an alcoholic. He has to be a total abstainer from alcohol. You have to be a semiabstainer from food, half on and half off the wagon at all times. A very precarious perch.

There are, however, three exceptions when we think it is OK to go ahead and cheat on your diet. In fact, we heartily recommend it. These exceptions are: (1) the day you win a gold medal at the Olympics, (2) your inaugural banquet when you're elected President of the United States, and (3) your 100th birthday party.

Of course, after all this preaching we admit that accidents will happen. Sometimes, for example, you'll inadvertently eat something that will turn out to have sugar in it. When you find yourself spilling heartily or registering a high blood sugar after such an accident, there's no need for self-flagellation and heavy mourning. Occasional *accidental* lapses won't destroy you. (In fact torturing yourself with frets and recriminations may do more damage to you than the dietary lapse.)

And, finally, to prove that we aren't as hard-line as we usually seem, we offer for your consideration the hog-wild variation (see For Concerned Family Members and Friends: If My Diabetic Son Goes to a Birthday Party or Trick-or-Treating on Halloween, Is It All Right for Him' to Break His Diet Just This Once?). But at the same time, we want to warn you that wild hogs can easily get out of hand and break down all barriers of self-control, and to assure you that June does not practice the hog-wild variation. *Ever.*

How can I stay on my diet when I'm invited out to dinner? _____

First, make sure that anyone who invites you to dinner knows you're a diabetic. That shouldn't be difficult, because people who know you well enough to extend the invitation will probably have long since been informed about your diabetes.

Almost anyone who knows you're a diabetic will ask what's special about your diet. An easy way to explain it is to show the person the answer to the question, "How do I plan a meal for my diabetic friend?" (See For Concerned Family Members and Friends). If you don't have this book handy, just be sure to mention the piece of fruit for dessert. You might add that any vegetable is fine, except that succotash and corn and peas and beans and potatoes aren't a vegetable to you, but rather they're like bread.

When you're actually eating dinner, do just as you would at home or in a restaurant. That is, don't eat more than you should just to be polite. It's always sound policy to wildly praise the host's or hostess's cooking as you eat your way through everything you can, while expressing profound regret that you can't gobble up every morsel and even have second helpings. Your words will probably speak as loudly as your actions, and the combination should satisfy the most sensitive of cooks.

How do I make it through the holidays without breaking my diet?

The holidays *are* a tough proposition. You have to develop a whole new philosophy about them as June has.

Remembrance of Christmas past: June was preparing a holiday dinner for friends. As always, she arranged a festive basket of fruit and nuts for dessert. Also on the counter was one of those fruit cakes that are actually more of a candy cake, what with all the candied fruits and nuts sugar-cemented together. This object of confection had been given to her by someone with a rather loose grasp of the principles of diabetes.

June eyed the cake with suspicion. "I wonder if I should serve that, too," she mused. "I can't imagine why anyone would want to eat such sweet gunk, but then . . ." she sighed, opened the package, and started slicing, "People who don't have diabetes are funny."

On the surface this may seem like the story of the woman watching her son in the Boy Scout parade. "Look," she shouted, "they're all out of step but Johnny." In this case, though, it's true. With the exception of a few highly disciplined, health-minded souls, nondiabetics are all out of step during the holiday season.

Remember the origin of holiday festivals? They were the few occasions in the year when peasants who ran around most of the time with hollow, rumbling stomachs could really fill up. Now, however, most of the people in this country aren't perpetually hungry. On the contrary, what a biologist friend of ours calls "hyperalimentation," or eating too much, is a national epidemic. The American public's overeating habits are bad enough the whole year round, but then along come the holidays with the atavistic excuse for overindulgence, and the scene becomes a dietary disaster area.

Revelers sometimes rationalize their holiday behavior by quoting the philosopher who said, "What you eat and drink between Thanksgiving and New Years's isn't all that important. What really counts is what you eat and drink between New Year's and Thanksgiving." Of course, this philosopher wasn't a diabetic. Diabetes doesn't take a holiday, and a diabetic can't take a holiday from health. So what are you to do?

Now, although there are gatherings where you won't be tempted by alcohol over the holidays (for the problem of avoiding alcohol, see Something for Everyone: Can I Drink Alcohol?) there's almost nowhere you can go where you won't be tempted by food, especially sugary food. In fact, we've noticed in teetotaling circles that cakes, pies, cookies, and the like are often toted out for the kind of indulgence that, if you did something comparable with alcohol, would produce a three-day hangover. Sugar addiction has been called the alcoholism of children. And we suspect that there are millions of adults running around who won't even sniff the cork of a bottle of liquor, but who are virtual skid row bums when it comes to sweet binges.

With visions of sugarplums dancing in everyone's heads and on everyone's tables, it's going to take all your ingenuity to stick to your diet, or as we prefer to think of it, your healthful eating plan.

Let's take the last first—dessert. It's not uncommon to find two kinds of pie plus fruitcake, cookies, ice cream, whipped cream, and candy being offered with nary a morsel of plain fruit in sight. But wait. There may be *some* in sight. Look at the centerpiece. It's often a lovely display of autumnal harvest fruit and nuts. Eat it. While others give in to their addiction to concentrated sweets, just sit there and nibble upon items you've plucked from the centerpiece or other household decorations. You should rhetorically ask the host or hostess, "You don't mind if I just have a bit of this, do you? It looks so delicious I can't resist and it's right on my diet." What can they say? It may give them a little understanding of what the diabetic diet is for future reference. You also may start a trend at the table. When others see you've had the courage to munch on the decor, they're likely to follow suit. Many people don't feel like a heavy, sweet dessert after a large holiday meal, but they don't know how to refuse. Show them how. (One warning: make sure the fruit isn't artificial before you sink your teeth in.)

If devouring the decor is beyond your powers of brazenness, or even if it isn't, a more gracious alternative is to bring your host or hostess a fruit and nut basket gift and when dessert time comes around, make your selections from that.

If the gathering you're going to is one of those where everyone contributes food, you could volunteer to be one of the dessert bringers and make something from one of the excellent and delicious recipes that are always given around the holidays in issues of *Diabetes Forecast* or *Diabetes in the News*. The other guests won't even be aware that they're eating a diabetic dessert if you don't tell them. (What they don't know will do them some good.)

Another way to avoid the dessert problem and yet still make the host or hostess happy is to take *one spoonful*. After all, if you've tasted the concoction, you can praise it, and that's the most important thing. It's also a way to make yourself feel less deprived. If you exercise total self-control every minute, you may build up some kind of dessert obsession that will eventually make you go wild and wolf down a huge hunk of mince pie. A little taste of dessert can do something else for you. It can show you that you really don't care for sweet gunk anymore. But only *one* spoonful, and we don't mean a soup ladle.

Let's face the final reality, though. No matter how careful you are at a big holiday dinner, you're still likely to eat more than usual. But there is one survival tactic. Exercise more than usual. Do as much of the cooking and serving as you can arrange to. If you're going to someone else's house, tell the host or hostess in advance that you'd like to help pass things, clear the table, do anything that involves motion. Most people don't realize the physical effort that goes into serving a dinner. A few Thanksgivings ago June virtually singlehandedly put on a family holiday dinner, and although she ate a good bit more than her normal diet, that night she had the worst low-blood-sugar incident of her life.

After dinner is over keep the exercise going if you can. Organize a bird- or star-viewing walk, a caroling session, a tree-trimming activity, charades with lots of physical motion, anything to keep the calories burning and the blood sugar normal. The nicest part about all these activities is that they're enjoyable in themselves.

By the way, an after-dinner activity suggested by the 1981 president of the American Diabetes Association, Dr. Donald Bell, is testing the whole family's urine or blood sugar. Since everyone will have had an abnormally heavy meal, it will be an appropriate time to see how their bodies handled it. Because there are those genetic factors to diabetes, you may catch a relative in the beginning stages and he or she can get an early start on controlling it before any damage has been done. It may sound a little bizarre, but it's a good idea.

Will vitamins and minerals help my diabetes?

This question is as controversial as the question of whether vitamin and mineral pills do anybody any good. There are doctors who claim that the only thing these supplements do for most people is give them expensive urine. There are doctors who have a go-ahead-and-take-them-if-you-like attitude. And there are doctors who counsel their patients to take vitamin and mineral supplements to insure that they aren't missing anything vital in their diet.

Personally, we both take vitamins and minerals regularly. We do this because, despite the assurances of the Food and Drug Administration and of the doctor-professor newspaper columnists, we believe that much American food is depleted of vital elements. We also think extra vitamins and minerals make us feel better. Whether or not that feeling comes from the head or the body, we can't say.

As for diabetics, in particular, needing vitamins: it is logical that even if diabetics eat a perfectly balanced and varied diet, their meals are limited in quantity. If, for example, you are restricted to one small orange in the morning, it's a cinch you're not going to get as much vitamin C as the person who can toss off a full eight ounces of orange juice. Consequently, even one vitamin C pill a day—say, 100 milligrams—brings you up to a better C level.

And the same holds true for the rest of the letters of the vitamin alphabet. As Dr. Joslin, founder of the Joslin Clinic, says, "To be on the safe side, there is no harm in taking one standard polyvitamin—a mixture of all vitamins—daily."

Two minerals that are often touted as helping diabetics by improving insulin usage are zinc and chromium. So far, though, we have found no studies that give any conclusive results on these two minerals for diabetics. Therefore, we favor waiting for some definite evidence of their benefits before loading up on supplements.

One particular need for older diabetics who take diuretics is emphasized by Dr. Stephen Podolsky. He points out that these drugs can cause potassium depletion and this, in turn, can cause your blood sugar to rise. He considers potassium depletion to be a major reason for non-insulin-dependent diabetics to be out of control. A diabetic on diuretics should, therefore, try to eat more potassium-rich foods such as oranges, apricots, bananas, other fruits and vegetables, whole grains, etc.

If you're on a restricted diet, however, you may not be able to eat enough of these foods to make up for the potassium loss. In that case, your doctor may have to prescribe a supplement for you. Although, alas, according to Joe Graedon writing in *The People's Pharmacy* (see Reference Section: Suggested Reading), potassium supplements are not always well-tolerated. They sometimes cause uncomfortable side-effects such as abdominal cramps, nausea, diarrhea, and "a terrible taste".

There are hazards to overdosing on minerals and vitamins, too, but most of these can be avoided if you don't take excess amounts of vitamins A and D, which can build up in the body. High doses of C can cause problems if you take a lot of it over a period of time and then stop, because that can cause you to develop a vitamin-C deficiency. Also, megavitamins taken over a long period of time can cause temporary liver damage in some people. (Your doctor can give you a blood test to make certain you're not susceptible to vitamin-induced liver problems.)

And finally we're glad you asked "Will vitamins and minerals help my diabetes?" and not "Will vitamins and minerals cure my diabetes?" We, too, have read, in books of vitamin lore, fables of how diabetics were able to give up insulin injections entirely after loading up on vitamin supplements and health foods. Don't give yourself false hope. If you have surplus money, it's better to give it to diabetes research for a real cure than to the vitamin industry for a false one.

Are coffee and tea bad for a diabetic?

Probably. Many recent studies show that drinks containing caffeine accelerate the aging process and cause headaches, heart trouble, and genetic damage. It stands to reason that any chemical that does all of that is not going to help diabetes. But what makes it a specific diabetes negative is its tendency to raise the blood sugar.

Caffeine is not just found in coffee (150 milligrams per cup) and tea (50 milligrams per cup) but in cola drinks (45 milligrams per can), cocoa (15 milligrams per cup), and even in most headache tablets (35 milligrams).

In that peculiar way the government has of legislating the use of harmful substances (ketchup is *required* to have sugar in it), cola cannot legally be called cola if it doesn't contain caffeine!

Besides the problems associated with caffeine, coffee has a few distinctive problems, the most disturbing of which was revealed in a Harvard University study which implicates coffee in cancer of our beloved problem-child organ, the pancreas.

If you are a devoted coffee drinker, it would seem good sense to cut back and/or switch to decaffeinated, which contains only five milligrams of caffeine per cup.

Certain conditions like high blood pressure, indigestion, and insomnia would make total elimination of caffeine advisable if not imperative.

Since some doctors let diabetics drink alcohol, why shouldn't they also let them smoke marijuana? After all, marijuana doesn't have calories or carbohydrates. _____

Even doctors who let their diabetic patients drink alcohol don't let them drink very much. They permit maybe one drink, enough to be sociable or to let the diabetic enjoy the aesthetic pleasure of a glass of wine with a meal. They never allow enough alcohol to mess up the diabetic's head.

When you smoke pot, though, no matter how bejeweled your roach clip, no matter how expensive an oriental carpet you recline upon, you're probably not smoking for sociability, or for aesthetic pleasure. You're smoking for one reason and one reason only—to get high. And high is the last thing you need to be, especially if you're a juvenile diabetic on insulin. With your judgment impaired, you can easily forget to eat. You can forget to take your insulin or you might be unable to measure it correctly. All this can lead to one form of diabetic disaster or another.

Even non-insulin-takers can get themselves into trouble while seeking splendor in the grass. Following a diabetic regime is so complex that it demands all your faculties in good working order. You also have to consider the "munchies," that condition in which a marijuana smoker becomes ravenously hungry and wants to, and usually does, eat everything in sight. Think how that could louse up your diabetic diet.

Remember, too, that smoking pot is still smoking. *Playboy* magazine once said that smoking, with its high cancer and heart attack odds, may be the big risk associated with marijuana use.

Finally, there are still a lot of unknowns about marijuana, more unknowns than knowns. Robert F. Forney, toxicologist at the University of Indiana Medical School, says, "We don't know nearly as much about marijuana as we know about cyclamates and birth control pills." As you may have noticed, most of the revelations about these two drugs have been bad news.

You already have one great complicator in your life—diabetes. Why compound the complication with a mystery drug like marijuana?

What should I do if I'm always too tired to exercise?

To some extent, that depends on what you did to get tired. If you're weary from your job as steeplejack or longshoreman, or if you're a housewife who's cleaned the whole house or galloped after a four-year-old all day, you've already had a great deal of exercise. Getting more is not that critical for you.

On the other hand, if you're tired from a long day of sedentary office tensions or sitting in the car, then you need exercise for more reasons than diabetic ones, and you should clamp your jaw and force yourself, at least initially. Just as the appetite comes with the eating, the energy and enthusiasm for exercise come with the exercising. Often the fatigue you feel at the end of a day comes from a *lack* of physical activity rather than from too much of it.

If you find yourself too tired to exercise and it's not a true physical tiredness, you may go to bed and find yourself too keyed up and tense to sleep. The next day you've got a lack-of-sleep tiredness going. Vicious cycle. But if you get out there and move those bones around, blessed sleep will descend upon you as soon as you hit the pillow. You'll sleep the sleep of the physically tired and virtuous. And you can hardly sleep better sleep than that.

Why do doctors always insist that diabetics give up smoking? _____

Smoking is dangerous for everyone, but doubly dangerous for diabetics. Inhaling cigarette smoke affects the blood vessels. Diabetes can affect the blood vessels. Both diabetes and smoking tend to narrow them, and narrowed arteries can cause heart disease and gangrene.

A diabetic has 2.5 times the normal chances of getting heart disease. A smoker has 1.7 times the normal chances of dying of heart disease. Put the two together and you have over four times the normal risk of heart disease.

A diabetic has sixty times the normal chances of getting gangrene of the feet. Again, smoking increases that already dismal figure.

A study done at the University Hospital in Copenhagen, Denmark, found that diabetic patients who smoked required 15 to 20 percent more insulin than nonsmokers. Their level of blood fats was also higher.

You might call smoking a kind of Virginia roulette for diabetics. So why are there diabetic smokers? That's a question we have no answer for.

Why do they talk so much about diabetic foot care?

It's that same old vascular story. Diabetes causes hardening and narrowing of the blood vessels. This, in turn, causes poor circulation of the blood. Since the feet are farthest away from that great blood pump, the heart, they get the worst deal. Poor blood circulation is also part of the aging process. So if you're older *and* diabetic, you've really got to watch those feet.

And we do mean *watch*, because if you also have a touch of neuropathy, you may not feel a cut, sore, blister, or ingrown toenail and let it go until it becomes infected. Infections are particularly hazardous because, combined with diminished circulation, they provide a welcome mat for gangrene (tissue destruction), which can necessitate amputation. As Dr. Arthur Krosnick, writing on gangrene in the March-April 1980 issue of *Diabetes Forecast*, said, "Its primary cause is neglect."

Here are the foot-care dos:

1. Wash your feet every day and wear clean socks.
2. Always dry well between your toes.
3. Cut your toenails after bathing, following the shape of the ends of the toes. Do not cut too short.
4. Wear well-fitting shoes and change them frequently.
5. Examine your feet daily for signs of infection.

6. If you develop foot problems, go to a podiatrist (foot doctor) and tell him you are diabetic. In fact, we favor regular visits to a podiatrist.

Here are the foot-care don'ts:

1. Avoid crossing your legs.

2. Avoid elastic garters or anything tight around the legs or ankles.

3. Do not use heating pads or hot water bottles on your feet.

4. Avoid smoking; it reduces the blood supply to the feet.

5. Never walk around barefoot.

6. Do not use corn plasters or any over-the-counter medications.

7. Do not cut corns or calluses.

8. Do not put your feet in water above eighty-five or ninety degrees.

If you need convincing to make you behave yourself in the foot department, the Loma Linda Diabetes Education Program offers the story of a man who didn't take care of his diabetes *or* his feet. As he aged and deteriorated, he lost his sight and all feeling in his feet. Well, it came to pass that one night, without knowing it, he knocked his watch off his bedside table and into his shoe and broke the crystal. He walked around on said broken watch for two weeks. Needless to say, he wound up as a guest in the Loma Linda Hospital.

We don't want to give the impression that older diabetics are the only ones who have to be careful of their feet. Although younger people generally have better circulation, they still can get into trouble, especially if their diabetes is out of control.

A young attorney stopped by the Sugarfree Center one day just after having been released from the hospital. She had stepped on a toothpick and her foot had "swollen up like a balloon."

She had had diabetes for seven years but had not been taking care of herself. As she admitted, "It's just been two weeks [the length of her hospital stay] since I've accepted the fact that I have diabetes." The foot problem, which had been exacerbated by her poor control, had turned her into a born-again diabetic who was devouring diabetes books, restricting her diet, starting an exercise program, and testing her blood sugar —in short, becoming a model diabetic, but that's doing it the hard way.

The purpose of these stories is not to scare you out of your wits. It's more to scare you into your wits. As Loma Linda's Dr. Charles Brinegar put it, "We wouldn't tell you these things unless there was something you could do to avoid them."

If you are a middle-aged or older diabetic, you should watch for symptoms of diminished circulation. They are weak pulses in the feet and legs; cold, dry, pale skin on the feet and legs; lack of hair growth on the toes; and toes that turn a dusky red color when they hang down as when you're sitting on the edge of the bed. Be sure to mention it to your doctor if you notice any of these symptoms.

It is possible to improve or maintain the circulation in your feet with a simple exercise. Lie on a bed with your feet raised above your hips. Alternate pointing your toes and heels toward the ceiling. Do this several times. Make circles with your feet. First clockwise, then counter-clockwise. Sit up with your feet hanging over the edge of the bed. Repeat the same maneuvers as above. Do this exercise a couple of times a day.

When you get your feet in good shape, walking a mile or more daily in comfortable shoes (runner's training shoes are good) can be of great benefit.

Is it all right for a diabetic to use hot tubs?

According to the U.S. Consumer Product Safety Commission, all people who have diabetes, a history of heart disease, or blood pressure problems should check with a doctor on the advisability of using a hot tub.

They also caution that nobody should bathe in a hot tub with water that is 104 degrees F. or higher, since water of 106 degrees F. can be fatal even to fully healthy adults. (Barbara, who considers herself a fully healthy adult, gets rather frightening nosebleeds after sitting in Japanese baths or hot springs.)

The preceding section on foot care explained that you shouldn't put your feet in water above 85 degrees F. or 90 degrees F. Since it's a little awkward to soak in a hot tub with your feet hanging out, it looks as if tepid tubs should be the order of the day for diabetics.

I have a bad case of acne. Could this be caused by my diabetes?

Possibly. Some diabetics report that they have acne when their diabetes is out of control and that it clears up when their blood sugar is stabilized.

Then again, it's possible that your acne has nothing to do with your diabetes. Many diabetics have a tendency to figure that every physical problem that appears from acne to Zenker's diverticulum of the esophagus is related to their diabetes. When June had chronic headaches, she at first thought they were caused by low blood sugar. It turned out they had nothing to do with diabetes.

It is true that diabetes, especially out-of-control diabetes, can cause a variety of minor and not-so-minor health problems.

Still, you should try to avoid laying the blame for everything on diabetes. Not only does this make you feel more depressed and put upon, but it may also cause you to delay seeking treatment for whatever your problem really is.

What kind of eye problems can diabetes cause?

Blurred vision is one of the symptoms of long-term, out-of-control diabetes. After the diabetes is diagnosed and brought under control, vision usually returns to normal.

When a diabetic suddenly has blurred vision or other strange visual happenings (June sometimes reports seeing a large spot of light in her field of vision), this can indicate low blood sugar.

Because of the visual changes that can take place with changes in blood sugar, June's ophthalmologist always insists that she have normal blood sugar when she comes in to have her eyes checked to see if she needs new glasses.

The changes in vision you may have with low blood sugar can be disturbing, but they don't mean you're going blind. Blindness is always a worry for diabetics because you hear so many horrendous statistics about it. Diabetes is the cause of eleven percent of the legally blind people in this country, making it the third leading cause of blindness. It is the number one cause of new cases of blindness.

The culprit in diabetic blindness is retinopathy. This is a damaging of the blood vessels in the retina, the light-sensitive area in the back of the eye. In its later stages the delicate blood vessels of the retina may develop tiny sacs that can burst and leak blood, causing a loss of vision.

This is one of the reasons your doctor always examines your eyes so carefully: to look for changes in your blood vessels. The retina is the one place in the human body where doctors can actually see and inspect the condition of the blood vessels. Not only is weakness in the walls of the retinal blood vessels bad news in itself, but the condition of these blood vessels reflects the condition of the vessels throughout the body. You see, eyes are not just the mirrors of the soul as the poets say, but the mirrors of the body as well.

Retinopathy is another one of the list of diabetic horribles that don't have to happen. More and more it is being shown that good blood sugar control can prevent retinopathy. In a study of 451 patients at the Joslin Clinic, only three percent of well-controlled diabetics developed retinopathy while thirty-one percent of the poorly controlled ones did. Another indication of the intimate relation between blood sugar control and retinopathy is that the Joslin Clinic discovered that those who take only one shot of insulin a day are six times more likely to have retinopathy than those on multiple injections.

Even when retinopathy does develop, all is not lost. There has been a great deal of success in treating it with laser beams. As always, however, the best treatment is to keep your blood sugar normal and not develop the problem in the first place.

What is diabetic coma?

What diabetic coma means is that your blood sugar is high—it may be well over 1,000. You have diabetic ketoacidosis. Your sodium bicarbonate and carbon dioxide level is low. You are dehydrated. Oddly enough, you don't have to be unconscious to be in diabetic coma. Only 15 percent are.

To define it more bluntly, diabetic coma is what out-of-control diabetics die of. In 1970, 37,800 American diabetics died of diabetic coma, even though death from diabetic coma has been totally preventable since the discovery of insulin in 1922.

To avoid ever getting yourself into this dangerous state:

1. Do your best to always keep your diabetes in control.

2. Never neglect testing your urine or blood sugar. If it's high, test for ketones, too. If there are ketones, call your doctor.

3. If insulin-dependent, never neglect taking your injection.

4. Whenever you are ill, check with your doctor to see if you need to take more insulin.

What is a remission? _____

A remission is a period when diabetes becomes less severe. For example, an insulin taker might find that he or she can keep in control on less insulin or on diet and pills, or maybe even on diet alone. Or perhaps a pill taker can get by on diet alone. Sometimes a remission lasts quite a while. Sometimes it is shortlived.

Particularly common is the remission that occurs in juvenile diabetes after insulin treatment begins. This often causes the parents, who are already desperately clutching at straws, to think their child has been miraculously cured or that the diagnosis of diabetes was incorrect. False hope. Diabetes is still there. A remission is *not* a cure and should never be regarded as such. Enjoy it while it lasts, but realize it will eventually end and don't be devastated when it does.

What is a brittle diabetic? _____

Brittle diabetics (also sometimes called labile or unstable) are those whose blood sugar swings wildly and unpredictably between high and low. They are, as Dr. Russell Poucher, a leading diabetologist of Orange County, California, puts it, "on the endocrine yo-yo."

The term does *not* apply to diabetics who have a lot of high and low blood sugar because they're doing a bad job of managing their diabetes but who try to excuse it by calling themselves brittle. True brittle diabetics are doing everything right, yet *still* their blood sugar plunges and soars for no apparent reason. The excruciating frustration and stress of this situation cause further detrimental effects on control.

For a long time it seemed that these diabetics were doomed forever to be victims of the vagaries of their blood sugar. Now, however, brittle diabetics can often be stabilized with a system of tight blood sugar control using home blood sugar monitoring and multiple injections of insulin, or with the use of the infusion pump.

Are flu shots necessary for diabetics?

They don't always work because there are often so many different strains of flu going around that you get zapped by one your shot doesn't cover. Still, we think they're a good idea. Flu can upset control of blood sugar for insulin takers and flu shots are usually recommended for older people. Put those two groups together and you've just about covered the whole diabetic population.

Since flu shots themselves can cause rather heavy flu symptoms in susceptible beings, it's sometimes wise to take two half doses at different times. June always does this with flu shots and with shots she has to take for foreign travel as well.

Who are some famous people who have, or had, diabetes?

This is a list compiled by the American Diabetes Association. (We suspect there are a lot more closet cases as well as a lot more famous people in history who were not diagnosed properly.)

Menachem Begin	Mary Tyler Moore
Jack Benny	Gamal Nasser
Paul Cezanne	Gary Owens
Bobby Clarke	Minnie Pearl
Ty Cobb	Otto Preminger
Andy Devine	Elvis Presley
Thomas Edison	Mario Puzo
Totie Fields	Ham Richardson
Mary Ford	Jackie Robinson
Tony Galenta	Dan Rowan
Bill Gullickson	Ron Santo
Ernest Hemingway	Richard Schweiker
Howard Hughes	Kate Smith
Catfish Hunter	Bill Talbert
Ted Kluzewski	Spencer Tracy
Stanley Kramer	JoAnn Washam
Nikita Krushchev	H. G. Wells
George Lucas	

A good group. Kind of makes you proud to be a diabetic; doesn't it? Now all you have to do is get busy and become famous so we can add you to the list.

Can animals get diabetes? _____

Yes. We personally know a dachshund on twenty-five units of insulin. If you think it's hard to regulate a person on insulin and deal with their low blood sugar, just try it with a cat or dog sometime.

Animals even experience some of the same peripheral problems that people do. For example, veterinarian-author Michael Fox says that dog food manufacturers often throw sugar into their product to act as a preservative. Doggone them!

FOR INSULIN-DEPENDENT DIABETICS

JUNE HAS ALWAYS FELT THAT DIABETICS WHO TAKE insulin are the real thing. In fact, in some of her more resentful moments, she sometimes refers to those who can make it on diet and exercise alone or on diet, exercise, and pills as "those fake diabetics." Of course, she knows in her heart that it's not true. All diabetics are the real thing and have real problems.

And yet even the non-insulin-takers themselves realize they have it a lot easier. To their minds the ultimate horror is often the idea of having to go onto the needle—a "horror" that insulin-dependents already live with.

As June says of herself and her fellow needle jockeys, "You've got to admit that we're the ones who are most involved with diabetes. In fact, it's never out of our minds (and it had better not be!). We have the needle and the daily injections; the constant lookout for insulin shock; the need to have something sugary available at all times; the problem of keeping medical supplies in stock; the expense of needles, insulin, and syringes; the precise food requirements, with eating too little as big a mistake as eating too much; the necessity of stuffing some therapeutic food down for insulin's sake when you're not even hungry; the inevitable snacks between meals and at bedtime; the every-other-month doctor's visits (and bills); the incomprehensions of family, friends, coworkers, and acquaintances; the isolation and apartness caused by being different."

Because of all this, insulin-takers develop a special kinship with each other. All barriers are broken down. Seventy-year-olds communicate easily across the generation gap with eighteen-year-olds, sharing their problems and their solutions, trading information, and gaining understanding of each other and themselves in the process. It's a close-knit subculture in which every member will leap forward to help the other in time of trouble. It's almost like a secret society, "The Diabetic Mafia," as Barbara calls it.

In this section we'll share the experiences and discoveries of the members of our Diabetic Mafia family in hopes that we can put a contract on your problems and send them to the bottom of the East River.

≡ THE BIG QUESTIONS ≡

Where and how do I inject insulin?

Insulin can be injected into the arm, abdomen, hip, and thigh (see Reference Section: Injection Sites). To make sure you stay within the proper area of each of these sites, you can order "Site Selection and Rotation" from Becton Dickinson Consumer Products, Rochelle Park, New Jersey 07662.

It's very important, too, to rotate your injection both from one area to the next and within each area. The above leaflet will also help you do this.

There are differences in the speed with which insulin is absorbed, depending on where and how it is injected. These are the most important things to know:

1. Injection in the abdomen is fastest—30 percent to 50 percent faster than in other areas. Next fastest are the arms. It also acts faster in places that are lean rather than fat.

2. Exercising an area into which insulin has been injected also speeds up the action of insulin. For example, it is recommended that you avoid injecting it into your right arm before a tennis match, or avoid your thighs, if you are going to run or jog.

Do I need to clean the skin with alcohol before I inject?

We hate to advocate unhygienic practices but we also hate for you to get all agitated and upset if you don't have any alcohol or an alcohol swab along when you need to take a shot.

For what it's worth, June never cleans the injection site with alcohol. One doctor told us there was a British study in which they gave 5,000 injections using alcohol and 5,000 without. There were only five infections in the whole lot and all those were in cases where alcohol had been used! (The doctor laughed and said maybe the alcohol irritated the bacteria and stirred them into action.)

When should I take my insulin? ___

Your doctor will no doubt have suggestions on this, but in general the answer to this question depends on how many injections you take a day. Most diabetics on insulin take one shot a day, and that one is taken before breakfast; usually, the recommended time is one-half hour before eating. For better control other diabetics take two shots a day of mixed rapid and intermediate insulin one-half hour before breakfast and dinner. Still, a few others, and June is by personal choice one of these renegades, take one shot before each meal. These three shots are taken one-half hour to one hour before breakfast and one-half hour before the other two meals. (The insulin is mixed rapid and intermediate except before lunch, which is rapid only.)

Of course, the actual daily timing of insulin injections cannot be all that precise, because life itself is so unpredictable. One morning you may oversleep, be in a hurry to get to work, and take your shot five minutes before breakfast. Another morning you may get an unexpected telephone call after the injection and delay breakfast for three-quarters of an hour. We've heard of even stranger variations from diabetics, like the man who told us, "Lots of times I eat breakfast and take my injection after I'm finished."

In the final analysis you have to work out your own best timing with your doctor so that you can keep your blood sugar and your lifestyle as close to normal as humanly possible. To understand how the insulin prescribed for you works, consult the Reference Section: Insulin Onset, Peak, and Effective Duration Chart.

What if I forget to take my insulin injection?

At least you'll know you're not obsessed with your disease. But if this happens more than once in a great while, you'll need to devise some kind of reminder system, like a nagging husband, wife, or parent. If you have small children, you can give them a penny each time you take the shot. (They'll never forget, but don't let them con you into taking your shot twice.) When it does dawn on you that you forgot your shot, be sure to take an injection immediately—maybe less insulin than usual, if you're well into the day.

Sometimes the problem is remembering whether or not you took the insulin. Then you have to worry about getting a double dose or no dose at all. If you use disposable needles (doesn't everyone?) you can look into the wastebasket and find out, if you empty the wastebasket every day. There's no doubt that a good memory is a help to a diabetic.

What if I take too much insulin by mistake?

Then you'd have to eat more than usual to satisfy the insulin. If you miscalculate and don't balance the amount of insulin with the amount of food you eat and your exercise, then your blood sugar may drop too low and you'll find yourself in an insulin reaction.

How can I get over my fear of the needle?

First of all, don't feel that you're more cowardly than anyone else. We've never met any people who enjoyed sticking themselves with a needle. (And in fact, we'd rather not meet any.) We have met several, though, who swore they'd never be able to do it, but when the golden moment arrived they found they could, as Lady Macbeth put it, "Screw their courage to the sticking place."

Most insulin-dependent diabetics who inject themselves— and many do it two or three times a day for better management—get so used to it that it's fairly routine. (We won't give you that nonsense that "it becomes like brushing your teeth.")

Sometimes people can inject themselves for years without being bothered by it. Then suddenly they begin building up dread again. If you haven't yet conquered your fear or if you find it suddenly reappearing, here's what you can do about it.

1. If you have the habit of worrying about the injection and how much it's going to hurt, instead picture yourself doing it easily and without pain. Positive thinking brings about positive results.

2. If you've been having someone else give you shots, start giving them yourself. Not only is this necessary in case of emergencies, but you'll reinforce your feelings of competence. You may even discover it hurts less when you do it yourself. We tend to tense muscles when someone else is taking a poke at us.

3. This may sound ridiculous, but it's true. June found that when she switched from one to three shots a day an amazing change took place. She lost all dread of the needle. Our explanation of this is that the more often you do it the less time you have to build up a wall of worry. You inject your insulin as calmly as you'd do any other daily routine.

A dividend you get from mastering your insulin injections is a feeling of power, an "if I can do this, I can do anything" feeling. You'll find you become a stronger person in every way.

What about automatic injectors?

There are a number of them on the market now, and certain people find they help them over the psychological barrier. Some injectors, like the E-Z Jector and the B-D Busher Automatic Injector, cost under $20, but are not very sophisticated or durable, not that a lot of diabetics don't use them with satisfaction. These can be ordered through pharmacies or directly from the manufacturer. Watch for ads in *Diabetes Forecast*.

There is also a very expensive ($795) needleless injector which uses jet pressure to spray in the insulin. It is called the Derata Medi-Jector and can be purchased with a prescription from the Derata Corporation, 7380 32nd Avenue North, Minneapolis, Minnesota 55427, phone 612-535-6765.

June has never had any fear of the needle and has always wondered why people would bother with any kind of injecting device. That is, she wondered until a Pennsylvania diabetes educator, Esther Shuster, wrote us and recommended that the Sugarfree Center handle a new product called the GT Automatic Injector (Figure 5). This is what she said:

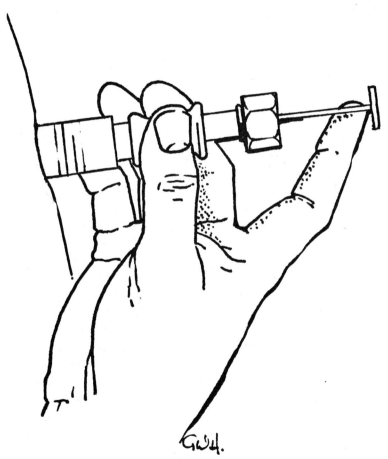

FIGURE 5   THE GT INJECTOR

I bring this GT injector to your attention because it has advantages over other devices. It is contained in one unit. There are no nuts, bolts, screws, adjustments, etc. There are no levers, triggers, or buttons to push, pull or slide. The GT has no adaptors for other size syringes. This device can be used by blind individuals when syringes are prefilled. The syringes, cap and all, are placed in the cylinder. This prevents bumps and damage to the needle. The device is easy to clean. There is nothing to take apart— nothing to lose or drop except the device itself. And the GT is sturdy. I have thrown it on a hard floor and it has remained intact. It can even be washed in a dishwasher.

Although I may sound like a salesman for the GT injector, I have no vested interest ... only opinions on helping the diabetic patients.

We got in touch immediately with the distributor and tried this little wonder. June fell in love with the GT and is now thoroughly hooked on it. Not only does it let her reach new injection sites and inject with either hand, but she finds it impossible to give herself a bad shot with it. It does not hurt at all and there is no blood. It is small and handy enough to carry around.

The GT is speed and depth controlled. No need to aspirate (pull back on the plunger to make sure no blood enters the syringe), if you make sure to choose correct injection sites.

Barbara likes it, too, because when she gives June her pop, June does not criticize her technique. We think parents and relatives would find it ideal when called upon to inject the diabetic. Nurses would like it for new patients. Since the needle is not visible when the instrument is cocked, fear does not have a chance to build up. For this reason it is especially good for young children.

The GT is available to fit B-D. U-100 (1 cc capacity), B-D. U-100 Lo-Dose (½ cc) and Monoject U-100 (1 cc) syringes. By the time you read this, it may be available for Monoject Lo-Dose also. In the works is an adapter to make it double as a finger prick device for taking blood sugars (like the Autolet).

There is one drawback to the GT Injector. It can cost anywhere from the mid sixty-dollar range to the high nineties and it is not readily available. If you have trouble locating one or if you can only find it at the higher price, write to us at the Sugarfree Center. We have it in stock and at the lower price.

We also have to caution you that in the beginning stages of production, quite a few flawed GT's were slipping through. This was especially true in the case of the Lo-Dose and Monoject models. We hope that by the time you read this the production problems will have been eliminated, but if you get an injector that doesn't work properly, return it immediately for a replacement. At those prices you should have a flawless specimen, and they *do* have a one-year warranty.

Incidentally, we've heard that some diabetes health team members object to having their patients use automatic injectors of any kind. In fact, some even refuse to mention their existence to patients, because they feel that an injector is "a crutch" and that using one indicates a denial of the realities of diabetes.

This makes June and Ron (both of whom use injectors) burst out in rants. June asks, "Is driving a car with an automatic transmission a crutch and does it indicate a denial of the realities of automobile transportation? No! It's just taking advantage of modern technology to make life a little easier."

Ron fumes that in using an automatic injector the only thing he's denying is unnecessary pain.

They chorus a final yelp of protest that nobody says that using an Autolet instead of jabbing yourself with a Lancet or an old insulin needle is a crutch or a denial, so why single out automatic injectors for a boycott?

Aside from the minor considerations of ease and diminished pain, automatic injectors can eliminate more serious problems. We met one young woman—a professional photographer—who was nearly blind in one eye and starting to get signs of retinopathy in the other. She should have been on multiple injections to improve control and prevent further deterioration, but she so hated the injection process that she refused to do it. Getting an injector made her willing to accept multiple injections.

Then there was an elderly diabetic who had arthritis in his hands and couldn't manipulate the slender syringes to give himself injections. His problem was solved with an automatic injector and having his syringes preloaded at the doctor's office.

How do I know when I'm having an insulin reaction? _____

Several physical and/or mental changes take place. You have to learn to recognize the signals.

> *If your blood sugar is dropping fast:* shakiness, sweatiness, dizziness, poor coordination, palpitations, hunger, irritability, and nausea.

> *If your blood sugar is dropping slowly:* slurring speech, blurring vision, confusion. You may be so confused, in fact, that you don't realize you're having a reaction.

One easy way to check on low blood sugar is to take your pulse. During a reaction your pulse will ordinarily be one-third higher than your resting pulse. (Be sure to learn what your resting pulse is if you want to be able to use this method of verifying reactions. To find out, take it several times when you are sitting around doing nothing.)

A little more time-consuming but decidedly more accurate way is to take your blood sugar with a Chemstrip (see Something for Everyone: How Can I Tell If My Diabetes Is in Control?). If you find you're too confused and fumbly to do that, you're almost certainly having a reaction.

Why do I sometimes feel as if I'm having an insulin reaction when my blood sugar is normal?

It could be that physical or psychological factors unrelated to your diabetes are making you feel strange. But we have talked to several diabetics who maintain that they feel better with high blood sugar and that when it's normal they feel as if they're hypoglycemic.

Most of those who experience this phenomenon have been running around for quite a while with high blood sugar, either because they weren't testing their blood sugar and didn't realize how high it was or because they'd just been sloppy in their diabetes care. You know the song "I've been down so long it feels like up to me"? Well, these diabetics have been up so long it feels like normal to them. Consequently when they start bringing their blood sugar down to where it should be, they feel unnatural. It's almost like coming off a drug.

But if you stick to it and keep your blood sugar in the normal range, before long you'll only feel right when your blood sugar's right.

What do I do for an insulin reaction?

You eat or drink something sweet that will bring your blood sugar up fast. (This always confuses nondiabetics, who are convinced that diabetics can *never* have anything sugary and may resist giving you what you need.) It's hard to know without experience exactly how much to eat. The more you weigh, the more you require. Also, you need different amounts depending on how low your blood sugar is. For starters these are recommended:

½ cup orange juice

1 tablespoon raisins

3–4 Lifesavers

2 sugar cubes

½ cup soft drink (*not* sugarfree)

After eating or drinking one of the above, your blood sugar will probably be normal within ten minutes, but your symptoms will last for half an hour. So don't be too anxious, overeat, and run your blood sugar up way above normal. (This is called anxiety eating and is a very common mistake.)

Richard K. Bernstein has people on his Glucograf system of tight blood sugar control use a British product called Dextrosols. These tablets are pure glucose, dissolve quickly, and are pleasant tasting, but not so delicious that you're tempted to snack on them. Bernstein has experimented with Dextrosols on himself and others on his program and found that each tablet raises the blood sugar around fifteen points. So if you take your own blood sugar and know how low it is, then you can take the exact number of Dextrosols necessary to bring you up to normal and not overshoot into the high blood sugar range. (Dextrosols are available from the Sugarfree Center.)

When I'm sick and can't eat, do I stop taking insulin so I won't have reactions?

That's a good question, as politicians being interviewed by reporters like to say. The answer is no, a thousand times no. If you have severe nausea and vomiting and can't keep anything down, you can sometimes reduce your normal daily insulin dose by one-half or two-thirds (if your urine tests are negative or blood sugars normal). But more often when you're sick, your blood sugar goes up and you need more insulin, not less. (Illness makes insulin less effective.) Sometimes your doctor (keep in touch when you're sick) will prescribe additional shots of Regular (fast-acting) insulin before each meal.

For sick days when you can't eat solid food the usual recommendation is to sip ginger ale (to control nausea and to satisfy your insulin) and to drink clear broth or fruit juices every hour.

Whenever you're sick, especially with the flu, a cold, an injury, or an infection, you have to watch your diabetes more closely. Take your blood sugar every few hours and/or check your urine for both sugar and ketones every two hours. If ketones appear, call your doctor immediately.

What is this insulin pump that I'm hearing so much about? _____

The insulin infusion pump (also called an "open-loop" system) is one of the most exciting developments in the world of diabetes. Some are calling it the greatest advance in diabetes care since the discovery of insulin; others are less hyperbolic about it.

Infusion pumps (there are several varieties being manufactured) are about the size of a transistor radio, weigh slightly under a pound, and most operate on a battery. You wear the pump on a belt at your waist or strapped to your leg (Figure 6). Pumps deliver diluted Regular insulin at specific intervals of time (every four minutes, every eight minutes, etc.). The insulin travels through a slender flexible tube and enters your body via a needle which you insert under your skin, usually in the abdominal area. You rotate sites just as you do when injecting in the old way.

The usual tubing length is about four feet. When you need to take off the pump to bathe, swim, or whatever, you disconnect it, leaving the needle inserted but capped. You can leave the pump off for up to two hours without raising your blood sugar unduly, especially if you're exercising.

The pump does not relieve you of controlling your diet in the same way you do with conventional injections, and you still must remember to take an extra shot of insulin (called a *bolus*) before each meal. You do this by pressing a button or twisting a dial to release the amount you need. Also, you have to test your own blood sugar three or four times a day to make

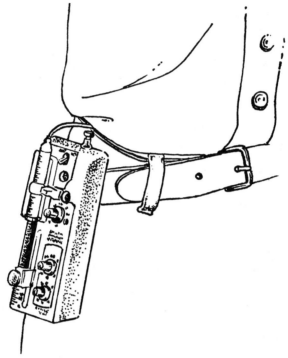

FIGURE 6 THE INSULIN INFUSION PUMP The pump is normally worn with its unobtrusive cover. We have illustrated it here without the cover to show you the instrumentation.

sure the pump is keeping you in good control. This helps you or your doctor to readjust the amount of insulin you give in the bolus doses, if necessary.

For ketoacidosis-prone and brittle diabetics who have been unable to get their diabetes under control in any other way, the pump can be a miracle worker. It was for one twenty-four-year-old woman we know. Theresa (Harris) Miller, whom we first met when she was a contributor to our *Diabetic's Sports and Exercise Book,* called us from the hospital one day in a high state of elation, because she was learning to use the pump and wanted us to come see her and hear about her new acquisition. The first day she was home, we did.

Terry explained to us that nine months after the birth of her first child three years ago she discovered she was pregnant again. Though her diabetes became almost impossible to stabilize during her pregnancy and everyone was predicting disaster for both mother and child, she did deliver a normal baby. But afterwards, she surprisingly became progressively even more brittle. Her blood sugar bounced from lows of 14 to highs of 999. She was in and out of the hospital until they finally gave up on stabilizing her blood sugar and released her, though she was still swinging between blood sugars of 40 and 600.

As month after month went by for her in this state, she began to feel too exhausted to care for her two young children, sometimes literally having to crawl to get around. Understandably, she grew seriously depressed, even admitting to her doctor and herself that she didn't expect to see her twenty-sixth birthday. The pressures on the whole family were tremendous. Something had to be done. As is so often the case with diabetics, Terry had to do it herself. She had heard about the pump and discovered a very special Long Beach physician, Dr. Michael J. Perley, who was himself a diabetic wearing a pump and who had a lot of experience in putting patients on them. She got in touch with him, and after an intensive physical and psychological screening, she was approved and put in the hospital to be taught the use of the pump. The rest is history and a pleasant history it is, with Terry's blood sugars now running 87, 105, 93, etc.

Terry remembers most vividly what her three-year-old daughter Tami said when she was talking to her on the phone from the hospital after she'd been on the pump a few days and her blood sugar was normalizing.

Tami: "How does Mommy feel?"
Terry: "Mommy feels good, *really* good."
Tami: (A long moment of silence, then with stunned disbelief in her vocie) "Mommy ... feels ... *good*?!"

Terry realized that her daughter in her whole three years of life had never before known her mommy to feel good.

As an indication of the difference the pump has made in Terry's life, Figure 7 is a copy of the announcement she sent out:

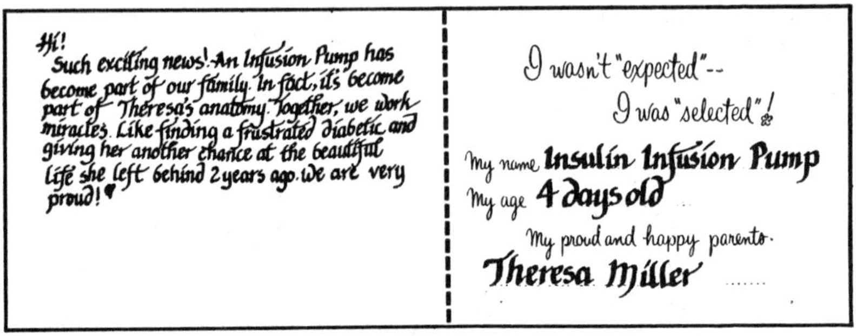
Hi!
Such exciting news! An Infusion Pump has become part of our family. In fact, it's become part of Theresa's anatomy. Together, we work miracles. Like finding a frustrated diabetic and giving her another chance at the beautiful life she left behind 2 years ago. We are very proud!

I wasn't "expected"--
I was "selected"!
My name Insulin Infusion Pump
My age 4 days old
My proud and happy parents.
Theresa Miller

FIGURE 7

Now Terry's only major problem is how to wear the pump when she engages in one of her hobbies: Tahitian, Polynesian, and belly dancing. Knowing her, we're pretty sure she'll figure it out.

Although the pump is a highly successful solution to Terry's problem, it is definitely not for everyone. For one thing it's still in the experimental stage. By the beginning of 1981 only around 1,000 patients were receiving pump treatment. There are bugs to be worked out—not the least of which is the amount of human error possible on the part of the pumpee. Some diabetics get soreness or infections at the infusion site. The diabetic's physician has to be trained in the use of the pump, and few are as yet. Not every diabetic is suited to the pump. As one pump user admitted, "You need to be conscientious, somewhat compulsive, and highly motivated. . . ." And as Terry says, "You have to work at it."

Some diabetics don't like wearing the pump, since it's a constant reminder to yourself and others that you are diabetic.

Terry maintains that wearing the pump is no problem. She says it's lighter than her husband's message beeper. In fact, she says that people think that's what it is and that you're an important person since you're wearing one.

The pump is also expensive both initially (around $1,000) and for supplies. Most health insurance companies will pay for it, though, because the only diabetics who go onto it are usually the ones who would otherwise have to have many a costly stay in the hospital.

Though nobody knows yet what the long-term positive or negative effects of infusion pumps may be, the short-term outlook is encouraging. In a study conducted at Yale University by Dr. William Tamborlane, the average blood sugar level in patients put on the pump dropped from 237 to 105.

And there's Terry feeling good for the first time in years, wishing that she'd gone on the pump months earlier, angry that nobody told her this option existed, terrified at the thought of what might have happened to her without it, and passionate in her desire that we get the message out to other diabetics who might be in her desperate situation. And so we have.

≡ SHORT SUBJECTS ≡

How do I take care of my bottles of insulin? _____

Bottles is the correct word, because you should have more than one on hand. The back-up supply should be kept in the refrigerator (not in the coldest part, where it might freeze, and certainly not in the freezer compartment). The bottle you're using (or bottles, if you use more than one kind) should stay at room temperature and be conveniently placed in whatever room you use to take your shots. Don't keep your opened bottles refrigerated. Not only is it unnecessary, but cold insulin causes more pain when injected. Insulin remains stable up to three months without refrigeration.

You should by the way always watch the expiration date on your insulin. If you use it after that date it may not be as effective. For that reason, you can't stock up on huge quantities of insulin when you find it on sale.

When June finds herself out of control, the first thing she checks is the date on the insulin she's using. If it's slightly out of date, she throws it away hastily. (Although she admits it usually turns out that the insulin was not at fault.)

It's perfectly OK to carry your insulin in your purse or pocket (in a protective case of some kind) when you're not going to be taking your injection at home. Insulin is pretty hardy stuff. You just have to be careful not to freeze it or expose it to hot temperatures (above 100 degrees). Treat it as you would a baby. You wouldn't freeze a baby and you wouldn't boil it.

When traveling you don't have to worry about keeping your insulin refrigerated, nor do you have to buy one of those expensive insulin carriers to keep it in. In airplanes don't put your insulin in the luggage you check. Keep it in your pocket, purse, or hand luggage, both because the cargo hold may be too cold and because your luggage may get lost along the way. If you're traveling by automobile, don't leave your insulin in a closed car in the hot sun because the temperature can rise to damaging heights. (Again the baby rule applies.)

Do insulin syringes and needles require a prescription? _____

This one's a real puzzler. The answer is that they do and they don't. In California, for example, most pharmacists require only the diabetic's signature, but not the doctor's. Some, however, insist on a doctor's prescription. The laws vary from state to state and the interpretation of the laws varies from pharmacy to pharmacy.

We've never tried purchasing this equipment out of state or overseas but June always carries a doctor's prescription in case the occasion should ever arise.

What causes those lumps that I sometimes get after a shot? _____

It could be that you've injected too frequently in the same place or that you're allergic to the kind of insulin you're using—or both. Try to be more conscientious about rotating the injection site and, if the lumps don't stop appearing, tell your doctor, who may change the type of insulin. For example, you might be put on pure pork or on one of the newly developed "human" insulins, the genetically engineered kind that is supposed to eliminate allergic reactions. For a list of insulins currrently available in this country, see Reference Section: Insulins sold in the U.S.

Is it OK to exercise alone if you take insulin? _____

It's always better to have a companion for safety's sake, as well as for company. You especially shouldn't do anything potentially hazardous like skiing or swimming alone.

Still, there isn't always somebody around, and a diabetic does always need exercise. There's no reason why you can't take a walk or jog or ride your bicycle or play a round of golf by yourself. Just be sure you never leave the house without enough carbohydrate to see you through. *Enough* is the word here. Take along a lot more than you think you can possibly need. Then you'll never have to curtail your fun. Here are dietitian Betty Wedman's guidelines for judging how much to eat before different types of sports.

½ hour bike riding, walking fast, roller skating = 1 fruit added before or during the exercise.

1 hour bike riding, running, walking fast, roller skating, basketball, tennis, racquetball = 1 bread + 1 fruit added before the exercise.

1 hour canoeing, skiing, swimming, backpacking = 1 bread + 1 fruit + 1 protein or 2 fat.

Dietitian Wedman suggests that dried fruit, nuts, sunflower seeds, and ready-to-eat cereals can give you a good variety of snacks during exercise. Many of her patients like a trail mix of small shredded wheat biscuits, peanuts, raisins, and chili powder. Then there are the old standbys of peanut butter and crackers, cheese and fruit, or nuts and fruit for mid-morning and mid-afternoon glucose boosts for lengthy physical exercise regimes like bike outings, swim meets, canoe races, etc. She does not recommend salty snack foods and sugar-concentrated foods for diabetics.

I've been told I should keep a supply of glucagon on hand. What is glucagon and how is it used? ____

Glucagon is a hormone that's injected in the same way as insulin, only it has the opposite effect of insulin. It raises the blood sugar. It's used to resuscitate diabetics who are unconscious because of low blood sugar.

Even if you never use it, glucagon is a nice security blanket. (It requires a prescription.) Just be sure whoever might be giving you an injection of glucagon knows where you keep it and how to administer it. And caution your family members or friends that if you're in insulin shock and unconscious, they should inject glucagon rather than trying to force liquid or food down your throat. An unconscious person cannot swallow and may choke to death.

For complete instructions on how to administer glucagon, see Reference Section: Glucagon for Emergency Treatment of Insulin Shock.

I'm always afraid of having an insulin reaction when I'm asleep and never waking up. Can this happen?

No doctor we've talked to has ever had a diabetic die from an insulin reaction in his or her sleep, except in one instance. The diabetic went to bed drunk and wound up literally dead drunk. What happened was that alcohol suppressed the body's method of spontaneous recovery. Normally, the liver converts some of its stored starch to glucose and that saves you. So the moral of this story is always go to bed sober.

We have also heard that insulin reactions are abnormally dangerous if you have heart problems. The moral here is to be sure to have a bedtime snack. But that is usually standard procedure for everyone who takes insulin.

Can I get a driver's license if I take insulin?

Definitely yes. We don't know the regulations in all states, because they're all somewhat different, but we do know that in

California the Department of Motor Vehicles recently made the rules more liberal. Diabetics don't even have to reveal that they have diabetes unless they're subject to periods of unconsciousness.

Is it all right to drive a car alone on long trips? _____

Of course. You must, however, always carefully compensate for the behavior of injected insulin. Doctors generally recommend that diabetics at the wheel eat ten grams of carbohydrate every two hours. This means you've got to tote plenty of food along with you in the car.

It should go without saying that when mealtime strikes, stop and dine. If you know there's a dearth of restaurants on the route or if you're particular about what you eat, it's better to take along a picnic meal than to risk having to delay your meal or stoke up on snacks.

How do I adjust my insulin when I fly and change time zones? _____

Time changes only occur when you fly east or west. Flying west to east, your day is shortened as you cross time zones. Going east to west, your day is lengthened. We like the system of adjustment recommended by the British Diabetic Association. This is what they suggest.

When crossing time zones west to east, if the day is shortened by four hours or more:

> For those who take one injection of intermediate-acting insulin a day—reduce your dosage by 20 percent (one unit for every five).

For those who take Regular insulin or a mixture of Regular and intermediate-acting insulin morning and evening—reduce your *second* dose by 20 percent (one unit for every five).

When crossing time zones east to west, if the day is lengthened by four hours or more, you will be having an extra meal:

For those who take one injection of intermediate-acting insulin a day—increase your dosage by 10 percent (one unit for every ten).

For those who take Regular insulin or a mixture of Regular and intermediate-acting morning and evening—take your usual two shots plus a small extra third dose of Regular (about 10 percent of your daily dose) before the extra meal you will be served.

The British also warn, "Remember it would be more hazardous to become hypoglycaemic [sic] than to have blood sugar which is a little less well-controlled than usual."

This all may sound terribly complicated, but in practice it works quite easily.

June never has any trouble making time-zone-change adjustments, since she takes three shots a day. On flights she simply shoots Regular insulin before each meal. (Warning: don't shoot until you see the whites of their eggs. June has sometimes heard the flight attendants scrabbling around in the galley and taken her shot only to have the meal not arrive for over an hour later.)

To make the time zone change easy and graceful, you may want to talk to your doctor about taking Regular insulin before meals but *you must practice doing it before you leave home.* You don't want to start monkeying around with your insulin dosage for the first time when you're on a trip and your routines are already disrupted enough to cause confusion.

Airborne injection tip: When you take an insulin injection in a plane, do not inject air into the bottle. If you do, because of the difference in air pressure, the plunger will fight you and make it difficult to measure accurately.

FOR CONCERNED
FAMILY MEMBERS
AND FRIENDS

THEY SAY THAT ONE PERSON IN FOUR IS TOUCHED by diabetes. That is to say, you have it, you eventually will have it, or you are a family member or close friend of someone who has it. Since you're reading this section, you probably fall into one of the two latter categories. And you have your problems, too.

June, in her more mellow moments allows that she thinks diabetes is sometimes harder on family members and friends of diabetics than on the diabetics themselves. She may be right, especially when it comes to the parents of diabetic children. For many of them their guilt feelings, anguish, and constant worry are exquisite torture. Parents often lie awake fretting through the night while in the next room their diabetic child sleeps—appropriately enough—like a baby.

Some adult diabetics manage to lay all the responsibility for their care on a spouse. In these cases it's usually—but certainly not always—the wife of a diabetic who learns the diabetic diet, prepares it, and tries to see to it that her husband sticks to it while he remains aloof and unconcerned. On the other hand we had one husband drop by the Sugarfree Center who did the blood sugar testing for his diabetic wife. He calibrated the Dextrometer, took the blood sample, read it, recorded the results—in short, handled everything—because she refused to have anything to do with it.

Friends of diabetics sometimes encounter the opposite situation. The diabetic doesn't want to impose his or her problem on someone else and so will hardly talk about it, let alone clue in the friend on how to help on a day-to-day basis or even in time of emergency.

It's never easy. In a sense you family members and friends are like insulin-taking diabetics who walk a tightrope between high and low blood sugar. Only the tightrope you walk is between not doing enough and doing too much, between being oblivious to a diabetic's problems and being concerned to the point of driving the diabetic—and yourself—crazy.

In this section we'll try to help you with your delicate and nerve-wracking balancing act and show you that although you're touched by diabetes, you don't have to be pushed around, pummeled, and knocked out by it.

≡ THE BIG QUESTIONS ≡

Will diabetes make changes in our family life? _____

Only about as many changes as moving a hippopotamus into the living room. Each looms large on the scene, can't be ignored, has to be worked around, demands a great deal of time and trouble and care; and you never stop wishing that someone would take the damned thing away.

But strangely enough, you can get used to anything, be it hippopotamus or diabetes. Eventually when people express shock and concern, "Oh, you have a hippopotamus in your living room!" (Or, "Oh, your child, husband, or wife has diabetes!") "How terrible!" you're surprised they even mention it as an oddity or a problem. It's just what *is,* a part of your life— and you're living with it.

Can diabetes destroy a marriage?

It can, of course. Some marriages are so tenuous that they can't survive any adversity. In such cases, if it hadn't been diabetes that caused the breakup, something else would have.

Diabetes can also strengthen marriages. When one partner develops a potentially life-threatening or life-shortening condition, this makes the other realize how important the previously taken-for-granted person really is. Working together to control diabetes can, in fact, bring a new closeness. We heard of a long-married couple whose children had grown and who had gradually become so consumed by their individual interests that they hardly had anything left in common. Each was running on a separate track. When the wife was diagnosed diabetic, the tracks merged as they headed toward the same goal.

Does a diabetic child disrupt a family?

A diabetic child can disrupt it or can merely change it, in some ways for the better. Disruptions occur when the parents are filled with guilt, anger, or both. We heard of a husband who blamed his wife for the child's diabetes and threatened to divorce her "if anything happens to that kid." Obviously, he hadn't heard of the new theory of the cause of juvenile diabetes, that a virus is responsible, just as for the measles or mumps.

Parents fraught with guilt can coddle and overindulge the diabetic child. This not only creates resentment and feelings of being unloved in any other children in the family but can be ruinous for the diabetic child as well. Diabetes can become for the child an excuse for dependence and manipulation of other family members instead of a stepping stone to strength.

On the other hand, psychologist Barbara Goldberg, writing in the November–December 1979 issue of *Diabetes Forecast,* emphasized that every family of a diabetic child that she talked to "mentioned that, in spite of, or perhaps because of, the illness, there was a special protectiveness, helpfulness, and a greater sense of family closeness."

This also holds true if one parent becomes diabetic. In American families these days we tend to be more than somewhat child centered. If a parent becomes diabetic and needs attention and care from the rest of the family, this develops in the children an increased responsibility and sensitivity to the needs of others.

In one family, the father, who had flexible business hours, spent much of his spare time chauffering the kids to their many and varied sporting activities and cheering them on from the sidelines. When he developed diabetes and had a need for exercise himself, the kids made it their business to see that dad got his jog every day and they took turns accompanying him on it. New responsibilities. New closeness.

What can I do for my diabetic child?

There are many things you can do. You can help the child accept the disease and teach him or her how to take care of it. You can encourage diabetic children to achieve whatever they want to achieve in life despite diabetes. But there's one extremely important thing parents sometimes fail to do because they don't know it needs to be done—that's to help them get rid of some of the terrible fears that diabetic children carry around inside and suffer over and don't talk about.

Dr. Robert Rood, a San Fernando Valley diabetologist who works with children and adolescents, told a story about a child at a summer camp where he was serving as physician. This girl was a model camper, full of fun and very popular.

Dr. Rood, in checking out her urine tests, discovered that her one shot of insulin a day wasn't doing the job, so he decided to divide her insulin into two doses—morning and evening. This worked fine. Her blood sugar returned to normal. But *she* became very *ab*normal—sullen, negative, picking fights. When he took her aside to talk she broke down and started crying. "I don't want to die," she said between sobs.

"Die?" said Dr. Rood. "Why are you talking about dying?"

"I know my diabetes was bad before when I had to take one shot. *Now* it must be getting lots worse because I have to take two. I'm going to die. I know it."

Dr. Rood reassured her, of course, and she became her good old self again, but he had learned something important. You never know what's going on in a child's head. You have to take the time to talk and explain. Be especially careful if there are any major changes in diabetes routines, lest the child interpret them as Dr. Rood's camper did.

Diabetic children also sometimes believe their diabetes is a punishment for "being bad." This gives them guilt feelings as well as fear that if they're ever "bad" again something even worse will happen.

And don't overlook the hidden fears and guilts of the nondiabetic children in the family. Younger children can get the idea that when they reach the age when the older child got it, they'll get diabetes, too. Each day to them becomes like the tick of a time bomb.

Guilt feelings arise when nondiabetic children have harbored some quite normal sibling rivalry evil thoughts, like "I wish Eddie would die," and lo, Eddie gets diabetes. They hold themselves responsible.

Parents must be aware of these dangers when the element of diabetes enters the family. Diabetes means there must be closer communication, more understanding, and more openness in the family. And that's all to the good.

How do I help the diabetic in my life?

Learn. Learn all you can about diabetes. Become a walking encyclopedia of diabetes lore so you can be an intelligent and informed as well as a caring partner. Notice we say *partner*. Don't do it all. Don't try to take over. Don't make the diabetic—child or adult—totally dependent on you. That's not an act of kindness. Diabetics have to be responsible for themselves. After all you can't be around every minute—and even if you can, you shouldn't be.

How do I learn about diabetes?

The same way a diabetic does (see Something for Everyone: How Can I Learn More About Taking Care of My Diabetes?). It's especially important for you to attend diabetes education classes and diabetes association meetings with the diabetic. Not only does this give emotional support, but two sets of eyes and ears absorbing the information make the program twice as effective.

If you have a diabetic child, we especially recommend that you join the Juvenile Diabetes Foundation (see Reference

Section: Directory of Services for Diabetics). Their primary goal is the worthy one of raising funds to finance research toward a cure for diabetes. But membership in that organization has the additional value of putting you in touch with other parents of diabetics with whom you can share problems and—more important—solutions.

Playing games is an entertaining and effective way for the whole family to learn more about diabetes, especially the complexities of the diet.

One good source of games is National Health Systems (P.O. Box 1501, Ann Arbor, MI 48106). They offer four games that are appropriate for diabetics:

> Soup's On: A balanced diet bingo game for up to fourty players
> Wheels: A vitamin mineral bingo game for up to fourty players
> Good Loser: A weight control table top game for two to six players
> Good as Goaled: A dietary bingo game for up to fourty players.

Each game costs $15.00

The Twin Cities Diabetes Association (5400 Glenwood Avenue North, Minneapolis, MN 55422) has decks of "Food Exchange Playing Cards" for $4.95 each. Along with the decks of cards are instructions for playing several games, many of which were developed by children at Twin Cities' diabetes summer camp.

Another way to learn about diabetes is somewhat unusual, but if you're up to doing it, it will increase your understanding of diabetes tremendously and also help you develop empathy for the diabetic. Empathy is better than sympathy. Sympathy is feeling sorry for people; empathy is feeling how they feel, almost getting inside their skin.

How do I develop empathy
with a diabetic?

You live exactly as a diabetic lives for a period of time. This idea was developed at the Diabetic Unit of the Queen Elizabeth II Medical Center in Western Australia, where they believed that the staff who treated diabetics needed to know what their patients' lives were really like. Volunteers for the experiment were required to take injections, using a saline solution instead of insulin, test their urine, eat the diabetic diet including snacks at the proper time, etc. These educators only had to "be diabetic" for a week, but some of them couldn't even last that long. The only one who was really successful at it just gave up her social life entirely and stayed at home catering to her diabetes. That, of course, isn't the way to do it. You're supposed to lead a normal life. After all, that's the goal for diabetics and that's what everyone else is always telling them they can do.

As Dr. Martyn Sulway, the physician in charge of the program put it, "They found out that having diabetes isn't a piece of cake." (Australian pronunciation: "pace of kaike.")

Barbara, even though she thought she knew all she needed to about the diabetic life, decided to try the experiment, because she'd been haranguing diabetics for years about what they ought to do yet had no first-hand experience. She did it, not for a week but for a month. It was a revelation. (It is significant that the night before the experiment was to start she had a nightmare in which she couldn't find the Dextrostix and a lancet broke off in the Autolet.)

Although she'd always bragged about eating the diabetes diet, she discovered that she hadn't been nearly as meticulous about it as a diabetic needs to be. For example, she hadn't always turned down *every* dessert. Also she hadn't had to be continually worrying about keeping the inexorable snack on hand for an emergency *and*—this irritated her the most—she hadn't had to eat when she wasn't hungry.

She took three injections a day. In order to have a little health hype out of it, she shot vitamin B_{12} instead of saline solution. Strangely enough the injections weren't as bad as expected. At first they were an interesting novelty, but before long they became just a bore. Occasionally and for no apparent reason the shots hurt, but most of the time they were relatively painless. The classic statement that "it becomes like brushing your teeth" didn't come true for Barbara, though. Since she's developing a periodontal problem, the tooth-cleaning routine the dental hygienist has her going through is actually much more time-consuming and painful than taking an injection.

Because she really doesn't believe in urine tests anymore, she took twice-daily blood sugars. (And to her surprise discovered that she may have a twinge of reactive hypoglycemia.)

She even managed to get the flu (not deliberately) and decided that if she really had been a diabetic she would have wound up in the hospital because her diabetes care program fell totally to pieces. This really brought home how important it is for a diabetic to avoid getting the minor diseases that go around every year, and it made her understand something irritating that June once did.

Several years ago in the library Barbara was complaining to a colleague that she thought she was getting a sore throat. June overheard this and, looking anguished, groaned, "Oh, I hope you're not getting a cold." She showed such concern that Barbara thought, "My, what a compassionate friend she is," but June continued, "because if you are, I might catch it, and *that* would be *terrible!*"

Barbara also developed a greater tolerance for the foibles and peccadillos of diabetics. She has always been aghast at reports that some teenagers (and even one diabetic celebrity) shoot through their clothes when out in restaurants. But one night during the first week of the experiment she was dining out with friends and suddenly realized halfway through the meal that she'd forgotten to take her "insulin." She didn't know where the restroom was and the restaurant was so crowded that it was hard to walk through. She did know that the "insulin" needed to get in fast so, . . . zap!—right through the old corduroy pants and into the leg.

One of the worst features of "having diabetes" Barbara found, was having to keep your mind cluttered with it every minute. As June says, it's as if you're always playing an intricate chess game on top of whatever else you're doing.

The *truly* worst feature of diabetes—the worry about hypoglycemia and long-term complications—can't be duplicated in a nondiabetic. Still you can learn an amazing amount. (Barbara's injection-giving technique improved immeasurably when she was giving shots to herself three times a day. Now when she gives shots to June in restaurants or airplanes, she has a much more delicate touch.) If you do this experiment, your insights will probably turn out to be different from Barbara's and more applicable to your own situation and that of the diabetic you deal with.

If I decide to pretend to be diabetic, when should I do it?

As soon as possible. Especially if the diabetic in your life is a very young child. We think it would be a great help to see that Mommy or Daddy can take the shot, eat the diet and skip the candy, and test the urine or blood sugar.

We had thought this playing at being a diabetic was a pretty wild idea that few people would be willing or able to try until we talked to a young woman who had been diabetic since the age of three. She told us that she'd had a terrible time giving herself the injections. She'd cry and cry, both before and after. Her older (by eight years) sister took it upon herself to take shots (saline solution) along with her, having races and trying to make a game of it. It made all the difference in the world to the diabetic girl in getting over her fear and loathing of the needle. She really appreciated what her sister did (especially in later years), and you can imagine what it did for the sisterly relationship.

Incidentally, even long-term diabetics love the idea of a nondiabetic's doing all the diabetes routines for a month. The ones we told about the Australian experiment (and Barbara's variation) all said something like "Now they'll realize what we put up with!"

June also liked having someone else taking injections with her in restaurant restrooms and every other semipublic place. She said it made her feel less like an outsider. People who observed all this injecting must have thought the whole world was turning diabetic—rather like the passengers on the flight to Hawaii when we were on a tour for diabetics. When the flight attendant asked, "Who has requested a diabetic meal?" twenty people raised their hands.

Of course, if the diabetic in your life is non-insulin-dependent, you don't have to go through the whole routine with the insulin. You only need to do urine or blood sugar testing. As for the diet and exercise plan, you should be following that anyway.

Why should I follow the diabetic diet and exercise plan?

It will help keep the diabetic doing it. But that's not the main reason. The main reason is it will maintain your own good health. There's nothing peculiar about the diabetic lifestyle. It's what we all should be doing. If you read the recommendations for good health from the Department of Agriculture and Department of Health and Human Services, or the American Heart Association, you'll see they're nothing more than the well-balanced meals with fresh fruits and vegetables, whole grains, no concentrated sweets, and reduced fats recommended for diabetics. The diabetes exercise program, too—regular amounts of aerobic exercise—is exactly what everyone should be doing, according to all fitness experts.

Actually, having a diabetic in your life or home is a tremendous boon. It wakes the entire family up to the best way of living and gives them an incentive for doing it.

It's particularly valuable when there are nondiabetic children in the family. If a sister or brother or parent has diabetes and the house is therefore bereft of junk food, they're going to develop healthy eating habits that will stay with them all through life.

Then, too, if any of the nondiabetics have the genetic gun loaded with a diabetic tendency, leading the diabetic lifestyle may well keep the trigger from ever being pulled.

And here's what may be the most effective inducement: If you have a diabetic spouse and he or she follows the diet and exercise program and you don't, you won't be able to measure up to your youthfully lean and vital counterpart. This can be bad for the dynamics of the marriage, to say nothing of your ego.

We feel compelled to warn you, however, of a built-in hazard when you're a nondiabetic in the company of a diabetic. That hazard is the old slip twixt the cup (and the fork and the spoon) and the lip. In other words, although you know better, you are constantly tempted to eat for two, and, alas, you often succumb to that temptation.

Here's how it works. The well-behaved diabetic is eye-measuring his or her food at a meal and eating right on the diet. You're doing pretty much the same, or maybe you're eating a *little* more, because after all you don't have to be all that careful with your measurements.

Then it turns out there are leftovers. They'll never be so tasty again. In fact, it would be foolish to try to keep them.

And you don't want to waste all that good food. Think of the starving people around the world. So . . . down the hatch.

A few hours pass and if the diabetic takes insulin it's time for a snack because he or she has to have small amounts of food at regular intervals to feed the insulin. As long as the diabetic is munching you figure you might as well be companionable and munch along. Your snack which, again, doesn't have to be so carefully measured goes down the hatch.

Dining out is even more tempting and hazardous. Perhaps there's a bottle of wine and the diabetic permits him or herself one three-ounce glass. Somebody has to drink the rest. It cost a lot of money. You can't send it back, and they don't have doggie bags for liquids. Down the hatch.

Maybe there's a really fantastic dessert selection and the dessert comes with the meal. The diabetic prudently says no. Two desserts go down the hatch.

When you and the diabetic are at a friend's home for dinner, your eating for two becomes almost a social necessity. The hostess has worked so very hard on hors d'oeuvres and exotic concoctions—especially exotic dessert concoctions—that she's going to be wounded right down to the bottom of her saucepan if *someone* doesn't lap up with gusto everything in sight and ask for more. The diabetic can't. It's up to you. Down the hatch.

If this keeps up, before too long that hatch of yours is going to be attached to a tub, a tub that is in imminent danger of sinking. This is especially true if the diabetic in your life is a relative, such as a sister or brother, with whom you share the same heredity. In this case, with your eating for two you could chomp your way into Diabetesland.

You have been warned. If you don't want that long and healthy life insurance policy the diabetic has provided for you canceled, you have to pay the premium. That premium is to exert the same self-control as the diabetic and eat for only one. Then close down the hatch.

≡ SHORT SUBJECTS ≡

My husband wants to think and talk about his diabetes all the time. How can I get him off the subject? _____

It's hard to find a middle-of-the-road diabetic. Diabetics either try to ignore the disease totally or they become almost obsessed by it. Those who fall into the obsessive category are at least better than the ignorers. They'll probably live longer and eventually outgrow their obsession.

As a matter of fact, many diabetics are only obsessed for a while, right after they're diagnosed. It's not surprising that they should be preoccupied when they first confront a disease that demands the constant attention and thought that diabetes does. Much of the diabetic's talk about diabetes at this time is just musing out loud as he or she tries to figure out what to do; whether he or she needs another slice of bread to make up for that weeding before dinner, if those funny feelings indicate low blood sugar or if they're something totally unrelated to diabetes.

One way that might tone a diabetic down a little is to become more informed on diabetes yourself. By showing your husband that you know something about diabetes, he may begin to feel that he can let go of his desperate hammerlock on the subject and relax and let you do some of the thinking for him. If the two of you have workable, give-and-take exchanges on new solutions to his diabetic problems, perhaps he'll be able to cut his personal, lonely fretting time in half and start to think and talk about something else.

Your advantage in knowing something about diabetes is that when he does talk about it, you'll understand what he's saying. Then the talking will seem a lot less like a foreign language you don't understand and, consequently, it will be a lot less boring to you.

If this plan doesn't work or just seems to feed his obsession, then you may eventually have to get tough with him. Tell him in no uncertain terms that nobody loves a monomaniac and that he's going to alienate everybody if he can't talk or think about anything but his disease. This won't be easy to do, especially if you have sympathy and love for the diabetic. Unless somebody sets him straight, however, he's going to ruin his life by thinking of himself as a walking case of diabetes rather than a human being with infinite interests and infinite possibilities who just happens to have diabetes.

How can I help my child accept her diabetes?

First, accept it yourself. Children are great little chameleons. They pick up the attitudes and emotions of parents faster than you can say "Jackie Robinson." If you have the attitude that your child's diabetes is a disaster and a loathsome burden, that's the attitude your child is likely to develop. If you take his or her diabetes in your stride, accept the restrictions of the disease, and work positively toward helping him or her learn how to lead a full life, you'll instill these positive attitudes by living example.

Incidentally, your question hit on the number one, foremost, important adjustment attitude for a diabetic—acceptance. It may be the hardest to come by, but once acceptance is there, all the rest is relatively easy.

If my diabetic son goes to a birthday party or trick-or-treating on Halloween, is it all right for him to break his diet just this once?

Think how many "just this once's" that would make in a year. Before long, just this once becomes an everyday occurrence and bad habits are established. Your son's health and maybe even his life expectancy are diminished.

It's hard to see your child deprived, when other kids are loading up on goodies—maybe it's even harder on you than on him—but diabetes is going to be with him all his life. Now is when the lifetime behavior patterns are established. You're *not* being kind when you let him break his diet just this once.

One thing you can do on occasions when your child is being deprived is figure out some way he can get extra attention. Attention is an even more satisfying commodity to the young (or the middle-aged and old, for that matter) than ice cream, cake, and candy. Let him pass out the forbidden food to others in much the same way that some alcoholics like to act as bartender at parties.

You can also give more parties at your own home. That allows you to present approved food in such entertaining ways that neither your child nor the guests will realize, or care, that they aren't getting the junk food of their hearts.

As for Halloween, the first decision in these hazardous times is do you allow your child out at all? If you do, and he comes home with a bag of loot, ADA Board member Netti Richter, writing in the September–October 1980 issue of *Diabetes Forecast*, offers some good suggestions.

> Why not help sort out the acceptable healthy foods and save a few sugary ones for handling reactions? What about

the rest of the candy? In our house the garbage disposal is a great eater of "nondesirable foods."

Knowing that resisting candy will be rewarded by an exchange gift at evening's end might make trick-or-treating less frustrating for a child. For example, exchanging the candy for a Halloween storybook at bedtime can be fun.

Use your own imagination to help your child stay on the diet instead of using your pity to allow him or her to break it "just this once."

Now, after having given the official party line, which happens to be our own opinion as well, here's a more lenient variation reported by a physician whom we respect, Dr. Lawrence Power, author of the syndicated column "Food and Fitness" and consulting physician for National Health Systems (publishers of health reference charts).

A colleague of his who sees many diabetic children and young people says that a number of young diabetics, especially teenagers, who don't want to be different and who long for the fun foods their peers get to wolf down, totally rebel. They refuse to follow their diets and as a result stay constantly out of control.

This doctor makes a deal with the kids. If they promise to stick to their diet at all other times, they get six Hog Wild Days a year, six celebration days such as Christmas or their birthdays or graduation day when, as far as food is concerned, anything goes.

"Do you know how high they usually kick up their heels on those days?" the doctor asks. "A coke and a hamburger or a hot fudge sundae. Big deal."

Dr. Power, himself, adopted the Hog Wild Day method with his adult heart attack patients. "Everyone needs a binge now and then," he says, "whether it's mint bonbons, Big Macs, or a cholesterol quiche. Something in most of us calls for a break from the routine. . . . There's room for the occasional departure for a holiday. It is the daily habits that get us into health mischief, not the occasional celebration."

Only you know your child well enough to decide whether the Hog Wild System would be a safety valve that would let off enough steam to allow him or her to simmer down to a good daily dietary routine or if it would only break down the already flimsy barriers against hazardous eating habits.

If you *do* opt for Hog Wildness, you should have a clear understanding with your child that the six days are to be spread out over the year and not clustered into an orgy week that could prove disastrous.

Should I send my child to diabetes summer camp?

Unless your child is the kind who would be miserably homesick and suffer psychological damage in *any* summer camp, we think it's a good idea—especially for younger and newly diagnosed children. We've had reports from young people who consider their camp experience as a breakthrough in understanding their diabetes and in learning new practical techniques of management. Even more important to them was the realization that they're not oddballs and that the world is full of other diabetics who are successfully coping with the condition.

It's a genuine comfort for a diabetic to be in a situation in which virtually everyone is a diabetic and the nondiabetic is the one who's peculiar. Barbara had this latter experience one day at the Sugarfree Center. June and Ron, both diabetic, were on the scene, as was our cleaning woman, another diabetic. (We practice reverse discrimination and only hire diabetics!) Everyone who dropped by that day was diabetic. Even the mail was all from diabetics. Barbara began to get the creepy feeling that she was the only nondiabetic on earth and that there was something wrong with her for *not* having it.

Summer camp is also a good way for a child who has perhaps been overprotected at home because of diabetes to develop self-reliance.

One major benefit of diabetes summer camp is for the parents. For a short while you get out from under the stress and strain of worrying about your diabetic child. You know he or she is in the best of hands and you can get away for a little R & R yourself. You need it and you deserve it. Stress works its damage on you as well as on the diabetic child.

Summer camp can also give you a chance to improve your relationship with any nondiabetic children in the family. They may be developing feelings of being less loved because they don't get the constant concern that the diabetic child gets. A week or two of exclusive attention can be a booster shot of security and self-esteem for them.

We have heard a few complaints about diabetes summer camps, including one from a mother whose already too thin child came home five pounds lighter and showing ketones, and from a young woman who was disturbed and disgusted by the wild goings-on with alcohol and marijuana in one camp for teenagers. But these are isolated instances. The overwhelming majority of the reports have been favorable.

What can we do if we can't afford the costs involved with our child's diabetes?

There is help available in the form of Supplemental Security Income (SSI). This is a federal program that makes monthly cash payments to disabled people "who don't own much in the way of property or other assets and who don't have much income." Diabetes counts as a disability. A child's SSI payment can be as much as $189.40 a month, although some may get less because of their parents' income and some may get more because they live in a state that adds money to the federal payment.

To find out about eligibility request HEW Publication No. (SSA) 78–11039 (*SSI For Disabled or Blind Children*) from your local Social Security Office or the office in the nearest major city.

Even if at first you're turned down, all is not lost. You can then get a copy of HEW Publication No. (SSA) 75–10281 (*Right To Appeal Supplemental Security Income*) and try again.

How can I keep from getting mad at my roommate when he's obnoxious because his blood sugar is low?

It's tough not to get mad. You're human too and sometimes you have a visceral reaction that you can't control. Just do your best to keep calm enough to help your roommate get out of the reaction, even if he fights you on it.

After the incident is over you'll probably both laugh about it. Once June had low blood sugar and became furious because she thought Barbara had eaten her dish of strawberries (which she had actually eaten herself, but couldn't remember). After her anger came despair, as she wept over her disappointment about the strawberries she had so looked forward to. With a baleful look at Barbara, she kept wailing, "You stole my strawberries." Throughout all this wrath and woe, she steadfastly refused to eat anything else to bring up her blood sugar because, "The only thing I wanted was those strawberries and you ate them." In retrospect, the incident seems funny to us, but while it was going on it was like a scene out of Eugene O'Neill. At such times you feel you're dealing with an insane person. (Of course, you are!) So never take seriously or bear a grudge over something a diabetic says or does when in hypoglycemia.

You have one big advantage in this situation: You know what low blood sugar is and can usually recognize it. This puts you way ahead of the average person. Think how people who know nothing about diabetes must react when confronted by your roommate's obnoxious behavior.

What am I likely to do that will irritate my diabetic girlfriend most?

Remember the Paul Simon song, "Fifty Ways to Leave Your Lover?" Well, there must be 150 ways to irritate your diabetic. In fact, if that diabetic takes insulin and you catch her when she has low blood sugar, anything you do, including trying to get her to eat something to raise her blood sugar, can irritate or even enrage her. (Some diabetics in that state have even been known to hurl food into the face of the person trying to help.)

All diabetics, even when their blood sugar is normal and even if they don't take insulin, have their pet peeves. You'll just have to find out with experience what they are.

We can start you off with a few tips, though. A diabetic hates to hear the same phrase over and over from you. For example: "Is that on your diet?" "Did you remember to take your injection?" "Did you bring along a snack?" "Are you spilling sugar?" —anything you keep repeating begins to grate after a while.

June, for some reason, gets furious when asked, "Do you have low blood sugar?" (She claims Barbara always asks this in an accusatory tone.) Her response is usually a garbled conglomeration of "How should I know?" "Do you see a blood sugar sensor sticking into me that I can read?" "Do you want me to stop what I'm doing and take my blood sugar; is *that* what you're saying?" Rant. Rant. Rant. She actually prefers to be told "You're acting weird" or asked "Why are you being so obnoxious?" probably because it's not the oft-repeated phrase that she's come to loathe.

Nagging, which one psychologist defined as "trying to control with criticism," is also near the top of the diabetic irritation scale. Nagging is not only irritating to a diabetic but it's also a futile endeavor on your part. Changes are going to be made only when the diabetic wants to make them. The best that you can do is to help her climb Maslow's hierarchy of needs (see Something for Everyone: How Do I Start Making All The Changes I Have to for My Diabetes?) to the point that change is possible.

Another thing that will bother your diabetic girlfriend is if you cadge snacks off her. Insulin-taking diabetics need to carry sweets at all times in case of an insulin reaction. If friends who are aware of this storehouse of goodies persist, like Goldilocks, in eating them all up, the diabetic can be in trouble in an emergency.

A far, far better thing to do is to find out what your girlfriend likes for diabetic snacks and carry something at all times for her emergencies (and your own snacking).

Probably the number one irritant for diabetics is if you don't make an effort to understand diabetes. Among her close friends June has some she's known for years and in whose homes she has frequent meals. All of them have supposedly read most of our books, and yet they still have only a vague idea of what she can or cannot eat. They understand little about how her meals must be scheduled or what to give her when she has low blood sugar. Since these friends are not stupid, she can only infer that they don't really care. A feeling that your friends don't care goes deeper than irritation. It goes into the hurtful wound area.

How can I tell if a diabetic has low blood sugar?

It helps if you know the diabetic well enough to recognize behavior that isn't normal. If a generally easygoing person starts snapping and snarling, it may be low blood sugar. If a decisive person becomes vague, that can be a clue. Fumbling hands, glassy eyes, slurred speech, perspiration on the forehead or upper lip, a dopey smile, an odd, taut look about the face— all can be symptoms of hypoglycemia. Just about all diabetics have some signs peculiar to themselves that you'll grow to recognize, if you're around them a lot and are observant.

Even if you know the person well, though, it's not always easy to recognize low blood sugar. We still remember the time we were talking to the Glendale chapter of the Diabetes Association of Southern California and told about one of our editors who said she could always recognize when June had low blood sugar "because she starts being mean to Barbara." We noticed a woman in the audience frowning. During the question and answer period she said, "My little boy has diabetes and takes insulin. Often, in fact, *very* often before dinner he's a holy terror. I can't do a thing with him. Could that be low blood sugar?"

"Oh boy, could it!" we chorused.

She was really shaken, because she had been punishing him for the misbehavior of his chemicals.

When you ascertain that a diabetic does have low blood sugar, take action immediately (see For Insulin-Dependent, Diabetics: How Do I Know When I'm Having an Insulin Reaction?). Above all, don't follow the example of the sister of a diabetic friend of ours, who, when she saw he was starting to act funny, looked terrified and announced, "You've got low blood sugar! I'm getting out of here!" And she fled.

What should I do if we're out dining in a restaurant and my friend, who is diabetic, orders all the wrong things for herself? _____

Diabetics sometimes perversely do this. Even June, who is the most careful and rational of diabetics, has occasionally suffered this restaurant aberration.

The best thing to do when you hear the diabetically inappropriate meal being ordered is *not* to screech and rant and embarrass your friend in front of the waiter, but rather to order a diabetic back-up meal for yourself. Usually when her meal is presented to her, the diabetic takes one look at it and comes to her senses. Then you just say casually, without any lectures or recriminations, "It looks as if my dinner might be better for you than yours. Would you like to trade?" The diabetic almost always will with gratitude, probably as much gratitude for the freedom from lectures and recriminations as for the food.

Naturally, to perform this little sleight-of-plate act, you have to know what a diabetically appropriate meal is.

If I mention my fiancée's diabetes in a restaurant to try to get her something special, like a substitute for sweet and sour pork in a Chinese dinner, she gets furious and says I make her feel like a freak. What can I do?

This answer is simplicity itself. You say to the waiter, "I am a diabetic and I can't eat anything with sugar in it. Could we please substitute pork with Chinese greens for the sweet and sour pork?" By claiming to be the diabetic yourself, you take the burden of asking for special favors off your fiancée's conscience, or pride, or whatever area of her psychological being is disturbed.

After you've claimed to be the diabetic for a while, maybe she will awaken to the fact that having diabetes is nothing to be ashamed of. She'll come to realize that for the most part, people in restaurants as well as in other walks of life are usually happy to help out with little problems associated with diabetes. This is an important step in her acceptance of her disease.

My son wants to play football. Is that safe for a diabetic? _____

There have been several outstanding diabetic football players. Ron Mix of the University of Southern California and Coley O'Brien of Notre Dame are just two. Many high school football players shared their experiences with us when we were writing The Diabetic's Sports and Exercise Book. (see Reference Section: Suggested Reading.) No diabetic evil ever befell them because of football. If your son's diabetes is without complications and in good control and his doctor doesn't disapprove, then there is no reason why he shouldn't play.

There are two good reasons why he should. Participation in sports, especially a physically demanding one like football, will encourage him to take superb care of himself and his disease. For a young person, the incentive to keep in shape for football is far more powerful than a general incentive to watch one's health. Once your son has established good habits during his football-playing days, there's a fair chance he'll stick with them throughout his life.

He should be allowed to play football for psychological reasons as well. If his diabetes keeps him from playing football, he'll get the idea that because of diabetes he can't do anything.

On the other hand, if he plays football, his attitude will more likely be that, despite his diabetes, he can do everything he really wants to. Which attitude would you prefer him to carry through life?

Be sure that he informs the coach and his teammates that he has diabetes and explains to them what they should do in case he has an insulin reaction.

And finally, do your best not to show excessive concern every time he goes out to play, even if you feel it way down inside your own pancreas. If you load him up with fears and negative feelings, you'll wreck his game and maybe cause an accident rather than prevent one. A football player needs a positive attitude above all else and so does a diabetic.

NOTE: One case in which we feel you're justified in forbidding your son to play football is if your family doesn't believe in the violence of the sport and none of the children is allowed to play it. In that case it would be wrong to bend over backward and let your diabetic son do something you don't let the others do.

Should I give my brother his insulin injections? _____

Yes and no. Yes, you should give them to him sometimes. You can reach injection sites he can't reach himself, unless he's a contortionist. This is a big help. Since a diabetic isn't supposed to inject within one inch of the same spot for a month, you can see how easily he can run out of accessible areas, especially if he has to shoot more than once a day.

Another reason for giving him his insulin is that you'll know how to give an injection. Should he ever pass out in insulin shock, you'll know how to give him glucagon (see Reference Section: Glucagon for Emergency Treatment of Insulin

Shock) which is injected in the same way as insulin, and bring him out of it.

But no, you shouldn't *always* give him his injection. He's got to be mainly responsible for his own insulin shooting. No one should be that dependent on another person. It's almost like being dependent on another person for your breathing. It's not good for him or for you, either.

We know a nurse whose husband is a diabetic. At first, he tried to wheedle her into giving him his shot every day. He got nowhere with her. She was as firm as Senator Inouye's nurse after he had had his arm amputated in Italy during the war. The senator's nurse handed him a pack of cigarettes and matches but refused to either open the pack or light the match. She explained, "I'm not always going to be around to do things for you. You're going to have to learn to do for yourself."

Should I give up eating pastries so my diabetic roommate won't feel tempted?

Admittedly, it's a little hard to sit there and wolf down a huge slab of banana cream pie, if your roommate is watching you like a spaniel. You both feel sorry for her, you feel guilty, and these are very digestion-upsetting emotions. Still, you definitely shouldn't give up your pastries for your roommate's sake. She's going to have to get used to being tempted and resisting temptation. It's similar to an alcoholic's situation. He or she has to be able to go to a place where others are drinking and yet not drink.

There remains, however, a question you didn't ask. And that is, should you give up pastries for your own sake? Pastries are hardly the nutritional dream dish for anybody, diabetic or not. And how is *your* weight?

How do I plan a meal for my diabetic friend?

Just remember that a diabetic has to stay away from concentrated sweets—sugar, honey, molasses in or on foods, and canned fruit in sweet syrup. Many diabetics also have to restrict the amount of fat they eat. Remember also that diabetics, especially those who take insulin, need a specific amount of carbohydrate in their diet. Just have something like bread, rice, or potatoes available, and the diabetic will know how much of it to eat.

That's another point to remember. Just as important as what is allowed is how much. A diabetic must eat limited quantities of food. Don't be offended if your diabetic friend eats with gusto and then suddenly stops. as if someone has blown a whistle. There isn't a bug in the food or anything. It's just that the diabetic has eaten all that's allowed. Don't urge him or her to have more. That's being cruel. The diabetic would probably love to eat more, and it's taking every ounce of willpower to stop.

A basic diabetic meal would be something like this: a mixed green salad; meat or chicken or fish; potatoes or bread or rice; a vegetable or two (*not* corn and *not* any kind of beans except green beans); and fruit for dessert (either fresh or canned without sugar.) Now, on the surface this may sound pretty bland, but any and all of these elements can be combined in something like beef stroganoff or bouillabaisse or chicken marengo or lamb curry. Just remember, generally, what ingredients you put into the dish and tell the diabetic so he or she can estimate portions. As for drinks, read the information on alcohol (Something for Everyone: Can I Drink Alcohol?). If you're still confused about anything on the diabetic diet, just follow the advice of all the sex manual writers who say, "If in doubt about what will please your partner, *ask!*"

If your diabetic friend is on insulin (ask!), then you should indicate what time you're serving. This doesn't mean what time the guests are arriving but what time you'll actually have everybody sitting at the table with food on their plates. Then, once you've set the time, *stick to that time*, no matter who hasn't arrived by then (except, of course, the diabetic).

What should I do if I find a diabetic unconscious?

Unconsciousness can be either diabetic coma, which means the diabetic has extremely high blood sugar, or insulin shock, which means it's extremely low (see Reference Section: Insulin Reaction Information).

If you know the diabetic takes insulin and sticks to his or her diet pretty well, then you can be almost certain it's insulin shock. If you know how to give an injection and where the diabetic keeps a supply of glucagon, you can give a shot of that (see Reference Section: Glucagon for Emergency Treatment of Insulin Shock). If you have a tube of Glutose (concentrated glucose) or Insta-Glucose (liquid glucose), both available at pharmacies, you can squeeze a little inside the diabetic's cheek. *Never,* under any circumstances, pour any liquid like fruit juice or Coca Cola down a diabetic's throat, as it could wind up in the lungs and suffocate him or her. If you can't do either of these things, then you can give a sugar solution enema. With any of these methods the diabetic should come around in about fifteen minutes. In cases where none of the above treatments is available to you, call a doctor or the paramedics.

If you know for sure that the diabetic doesn't take insulin and/or doesn't follow the diet or take care of him or herself, then it's probably a diabetic coma, the result of long-range diabetic misbehavior. In this case, call the doctor or an ambulance immediately. There's nothing much you can do in this kind of a crisis. Only a hospital can help now.

If you have no idea whether you're dealing with insulin shock or diabetic coma, treat for insulin shock. If it's diabetic coma, the diabetic already has so much sugar floating through his or her system that a little more isn't going to make all that much difference. And if it *is* insulin shock, your quick treatment could be a lifesaver. A person in good health will eventually come out of insulin shock spontaneously, but for someone with a heart condition the shock could be life threatening.

Should I marry a diabetic? _____

That, like the decision to marry at all, has ultimately to be your own decision, as you undoubtedly well know. The probable reason for asking this is that you're concerned about the problems your potential mate's diabetes might cause in the future.

It's wise to think about these possible problems now rather than later. As diabetes teaching nurse, Diane Victor, said to a young man who was complaining about some aspect of his wife's diabetes and shirking his responsibility for helping to deal with it, "Look, you knew she was diabetic when you married her. You signed on for the duration. Shape up."

Diabetes is never problem free, as we've made clear in this book and as you have probably already personally observed if you have a close relationship with a diabetic. Diabetes care takes time, time you would prefer to spend on more entertaining activities. Diabetes care takes money, money you would prefer to spend on other things. Diabetes can make having children more difficult, hazardous, and—again—more expensive than normal. And diabetes if not cared for properly and controlled, eventually can cause debilitating complications and an earlier death.

But all of this doesn't mean you should give back (or take back) the engagement ring. Marriage is full of risks. You could marry a flawless specimen bearing a doctor's certificate of perfect health and the day after your wedding he or she or even *you* could get in an accident that paralyzed everything south of the earlobes. We have a friend whose apparently healthy wife developed multiple sclerosis in the first year they were married.

There are no guarantees in life. When you get married, the old "for better or for worse; in sickness and in health" still holds true. Realistically considered, diabetes, if well controlled, is one of the lesser worses and healthier sicknesses, and knowing about it in advance gives you a chance to learn and prepare and adjust.

In the final analysis we believe that love conquers all. By this we don't mean the short-lived romantic love that turns your mind to irrational (but delicious) mush. No, we're referring to the enduring, day-to-day-growing love that comes from living through and living with problems together and helping each other play out whatever hands you may be dealt, trying to turn a losing game into a winning one.

Just ask Theresa Miller (see For Insulin-Dependent Diabetics: What Is This Insulin Pump That I'm Hearing So Much About?), and her husband, Steve, how their struggles with her wildly brittle diabetes and the one difficult and one near-impossible pregnancy strengthened their love and appreciation for each other.

THE LAST WORD

REFERENCE SECTION

IN THE LOS ANGELES VALLEY COLLEGE LIBRARY, where we work, students often approach the Reference Desk with the hesitant opening gambit of "This may be a stupid question, but . . ."

Since we don't consider any question stupid if there is something you want to know or something you don't understand, we made a special sign to reassure the students who hesitate to ask—and those who never ask at all.

We hope that until the day they find the answer to the ultimate question about diabetes, you'll keep asking questions. Ask doctors, ask nurses, ask dietitians, ask sociologists and psychologists, ask other diabetics, ask us, and above all, ask yourself until you find all the answers you need to lead an exciting, healthy, happy, productive life.

Remember, as our library sign put it,

There Is No Such Thing As a Stupid Question.

DIRECTORY OF SERVICES
FOR DIABETICS

American Association of Diabetes Educators
North Woodbury Road, Box 56
Pitman, NJ 08071
Write for information on diabetes-education programs in your
area.

American Diabetes Association
2 Park Avenue
New York, NY 10016
Write for the address of your local chapter if it is not listed in
your phone book.

American Dietetic Association
430 North Michigan Avenue
Chicago, IL 60611
Can provide names of qualified dietitians in your area.

Ames Division
Miles Laboratories, Inc.
P.O. Box 70
Elkhart, IN 46515
Dextrostix, Dextrometer, Glucometer, urine tests, ketone tests,
Clinilog II urine testing record book.

Becton Dickinson Consumer Products
P.O. Box 5000
Rochelle Park, NJ 07662
B-D insulin syringes.

Bio-Dynamics
9115 Hague Road, P.O. Box 50100
Indianapolis, IN 46250
Chemstrips bG, StatTek Photometer, StatTek Glucose Test
Strips.

Consulting Nutritionists
A Practice Group of the American Dietetic Association
Virginia Bayles, R.D.
Membership Secretary/Treasurer
5018 Indigo
Houston, TX 77096
>Can provide names of qualified dietitians in private practice.

Eli Lilly and Company
Medical Department
307 East McCarty Street, P. O. Box 618
Indianapolis, IN 46206
>Insulin, Tes-Tape.

Joslin Clinic
15 Joslin Road
Boston, MA 02215
>The United States oldest and most reknown center of diabetes education, treatment, and research.

Juvenile Diabetes Foundation
23 East 26th Street
New York, NY 10010
>A national group whose objective is to fund research aimed at curing diabetes and preventing its complications. Information, educational programs, and meetings for diabetic children and young people and their families. Write for address of your local chapter.

Monoject
Division of Sherwood Medical
1831 Olive Street
St. Louis, MO 63103
>Monoject insulin syringes, Monolet Lancets, insulin travel kit, scale magnifier for insulin syringes.

Nordisk
7315 Wisconsin Avenue
Bethesda, MD 20014
  Pure pork insulins.

Novo Laboratories, Incorporated
59 Danbury Road
Wilton, CT 06897
  Purified insulins.

Sugarfree Center for Diabetics
5623 Matilija Avenue, P.O. Box 2166
Van Nuys, CA 91401
  A mail order service featuring hard-to-find diabetes books, blood sugar testing materials, and new self-care products. Write for free brochure. June Biermann and Barbara Toohey, directors.

EXCHANGE SYSTEM
MEAL PLANS

It is important to eat consistent amounts of carbohydrates at regular times throughout the day. Children with diabetes mellitus may need three meals with three snacks daily to provide a steady supply of carbohydrates. Children usually take more milk than adults and unless there is some special consideration, skim milk is suggested as a routine.

Bedtime snacks are commonly used by both adult and child diabetics. They should supply both protein and carbohydrate.

Special Note: The Committee on Food and Nutrition of the American Diabetes Association has recommended since 1979 that dietary sources of fat high in saturated fatty acids and high in cholesterol should be restricted. The Committee also recommends that natural foods containing unrefined carbohydrate (fiber) should be substituted for highly refined carbohydrates that are low in fiber, and that attention be paid to the amount of salt in the diet.

The chart above is adapted from the National Health System's picture poster "The New Diabetes Unit." It is reprinted by permission of Lawrence Power, M.D. and Adria Myeroff, R.D.

Daily Calories:		1000	1200	1500	1800 (Child)	1800	2000	2200	2500 (Child)	2500
(Meat) Exchanges	Breakfast	1	1	1	0	1	1	1	1	2
	Lunch	2	2	2	1	2	3	3	2	3
	Dinner	2	3	3	2	3	3	3	2	3
	Bedtime	0	0	0	1	1	1	1	1	2
Vegetable Exchanges	Breakfast	0	0	0	0	0	0	0	0	0
	Lunch	1	1	1	1	1	1	1	1	1
	Dinner	1	1	2	1	2	2	2	1	2
	Bedtime	0	0	0	0	0	0	0	0	0
Fruit Exchanges	Breakfast	1	1	1	1	1	1	2	2	2
	Lunch	1	1	1	1	1	2	2	3	3
	Dinner	1	1	1	1	2	2	2	2	2
	Bedtime	0	0	1	1	1	1	1	0	1
Bread Exchanges	Breakfast	1	1	1	2	2	2	3	2	3
	Lunch	1	2	2	2	2	3	3	3	3
	Dinner	1	1	2	2	2	2	3	3	4
	Bedtime	0	1	1	2	2	2	2	2	2
Fat Exchanges	Breakfast	1	1	1	2	2	2	2	2	2
	Lunch	0	0	1	2	1	1	2	2	2
	Dinner	1	1	2	2	2	2	2	2	2
	Bedtime	0	0	0	1	0	0	0	1	1
Skim Milk		2	2	3	3	3	3	3	4	3

BRAND-NAME
EXCHANGES

In the past two years, the magazine *Better Homes and Gardens* has published lists of diabetic exchanges three times. The following list includes foods from all three lists, plus a few others. Both *Better Homes and Gardens* and the manufacturers listed cooperated in supplying us with the figures below.

For information about the carbohydrate, protein, fat, and calorie content of these and other manufactured foods, look at the nutrition labels or write to the manufacturers.

BRAND-NAME EXCHANGES

Main Dishes	Serving Size	Exchanges per Serving	Calories per Serving*
Betty Crocker			
chili-tomato Hamburger Helper mix	1/5 package	2 bread + 1/2 fat	140
hamburger stew Hamburger Helper mix	1/5 package	1 1/2 bread	110
lasagna Hamburger Helper mix	1/5 package	2 bread	150
spaghetti Hamburger Helper mix	1/5 package	2 bread	150
Dinty Moore®			
beef stew	7 1/2 ounces	1/2 bread + 1 1/2 low-fat meat + 1 vegetable + 1 fat	180
vegetable stew	7 1/2 ounces	1 bread + 1 vegetable + 2 fat	160
noodles 'n chicken	7 1/2 ounces	1 bread + 1 low-fat meat + 2 fat	215
Heinz			
vegetarian beans in tomato sauce	8 ounces	1 vegetable + 1 fruit + 2 bread	220
beef stew	7 1/4 ounces	1 vegetable + 1 bread + 1 low-fat meat + 1 fat	200
chicken stew with dumplings	7 1/4 ounces	1 vegetable + 1 bread + 1 low-fat meat + 1 fat	200
macaroni in cheese sauce	7 1/2 ounces	1 1/2 bread + 1 low-fat meat + 1/2 fat	180
spaghetti with meat sauce	7 1/4 ounces	1 vegetable + 1 bread + 1/2 low-fat meat + 1 fat	170

Hormel			
noodles 'n beef	7½ ounces	1 bread + 1 low-fat meat + 2 fat	240
spaghetti and meatballs	7½ ounces	1½ bread + ½ low-fat meat + 1 fat	170
beef goulash	7½ ounces	1 bread + 1½ low-fat meat + ½ vegetable + 2 fat	240
Kraft			
macaroni and cheese dinner mix (prepared)	¾ cup	2 bread + ½ high-fat meat + 2 fat	280
American-style spaghetti dinner mix (prepared)	1 cup	3 bread + 1 fat	260
cheese pizza mix	¼ box	2½ bread + 1 high-fat meat	250
sausage pizza mix	¼ box	2½ bread + 1 high-fat meat + ½ fat	280
Mrs. Paul's			
frozen deviled crab cakes	1 cake	1 high-fat meat + 1 bread	220
frozen fish sticks	4 sticks	1 medium-fat meat + 1 bread	210
Swanson®			
(canned products only)			
boned chicken or turkey	2½ ounces	2 low-fat meat	110
chicken spread	1 ounce	1 low-fat meat	70
chunk white chicken	2½ ounces	2 low-fat meat	110
beef stew	7½ ounces	1 vegetable + 1 bread + 1 low-fat meat + 1 fat	190
chicken stew	7½ ounces	1 vegetable + 1 bread + 1 low-fat meat + 1 fat	180
chicken a la king	5¼ ounces	½ bread + 2 low-fat meat + 1 fat	190
chicken and dumplings	7½ ounces	1 bread + 2 low-fat meat + 1 fat	230
chili con carne with beans	7¾ ounces	2 bread + 2 low-fat meat + 1½ fat	310

BRAND-NAME EXCHANGES *(continued)*

Meal Accompaniments	Serving Size	Exchanges per Serving	Calories per Serving*
Birds Eye			
frozen French-style green beans with mushrooms	3 ounces	1 vegetable	30
frozen mixed vegetables with onion sauce	2.6 ounces	2 vegetable + 1 fat	110
frozen green peas and onions	3.3 ounces	2 vegetable	60
frozen Bavarian-style beans with spaetzle	3.3 ounces	2 vegetable	50
frozen Chinese-style vegetables	3.3 ounces	1 vegetable	25
frozen Danish-style vegetables	3.3 ounces	1 vegetable	45
frozen Italian-style vegetables	3.3 ounces	½ bread	60
frozen Japanese-style vegetables	3.3 ounces	1 vegetable	40
Betty Crocker			
packaged noodles almondine mix (prepared)	¼ package	2 bread + 2 fat	240
packaged noodles Romanoff mix (prepared)	¼ package	1 bread + ½ milk + 2 fat	230

218

	Serving Size	Exchanges per Serving	Calories per Serving
instant mashed potato buds	1/3 cup	1½ bread	130
dry scalloped potato mix	1/8 package	1½ bread	150
dry hash brown potato mix	1/8 package	1½ bread	150
Minute packaged precooked rice mixes (beef-flavored, Spanish, chicken-flavored, fried)	½ cup	2 bread + 1 fat	170
Stove Top packaged stuffing mix (prepared with butter)	½ cup	1½ bread + 2 fat	170

Soups	Serving Size	Exchanges per Serving	Calories per Serving*
Campbell's® Condensed (prepared with water)			
cheddar cheese	11 ounces	1 milk + 3 fat	200
chicken, cream of	10 ounces	½ bread + 2 fat	140
chicken noodle	10 ounces	1 Bread	90
chicken with rice	10 ounces	1 Bread	80
clam chowder, Manhattan	10 ounces	1 bread + ½ fat	100
clam chowder, New England (prepared with nonfat milk)	10 ounces	½ milk + 1 bread + 1 low-fat meat	120
minestrone	10 ounces	1 bread + ½ fat	110

BRAND-NAME EXCHANGES *(continued)*

Soups	Serving Size	Exchanges per Serving	Calories per Serving*
mushroom, cream of	10 ounces	1 bread + 2 fat	150
tomato	10 ounces	1 vegetable + 1 bread	110
vegetable	10 ounces	1 vegetable + 1 bread	100
vegetable beef	10 ounces	½ bread + 1 low-fat meat	90
vegetarian vegetable	10 ounces	1 bread	90
chunky chicken (undiluted)	9½ ounces	1 vegetable + 1 bread + 2 low-fat meat	200
chunky chili beef (undiluted)	9½ ounces	2 bread + 2 low-fat meat	260
chunky sirloin burger (undiluted)	9½ ounces	1 vegetable + 1 bread + 1 low-fat meat + 1 fat	210
Lipton Cup-a-Soup (prepared)			
1-serving-size dry cream-style chicken	6 ounces	⅔ bread + 1 fat	80
1-serving-size cream of mushroom	6 ounces	⅔ bread + 1 fat	80
1-serving-size beef-flavored noodle	6 ounces	½ bread	35
1-serving-size chicken noodle with meat	6 ounces	½ bread	45
1-serving-size green pea	6 ounces	1½ bread + ½ low-fat meat	120

1-serving-size cream of tomato	6 ounces	1 bread + ½ fat	70
1-serving-size spring vegetable	6 ounces	2 vegetable	45

Lipton Soup Mixes

1-serving size onion**	6 ounces	1 vegetable	35
1-serving size beefy-onion**	6 ounces	1 vegetable	30

Nestle Souptime (prepared)

1-serving-size chicken noodle	6 ounces	½ bread	30
1-serving-size beef noodle	6 ounces	½ bread	30
1-serving-size cream of chicken	6 ounces	⅔ bread + 1 fat	100
1-serving-size tomato	6 ounces	1 bread	70
1-serving-size French onion	6 ounces	1 vegetable	20
1-serving-size green pea	6 ounces	1 bread + ½ low-fat meat	70
1-serving-size mushroom	6 ounces	⅔ bread + 1 fat	80
1-serving-size cream of vegetable	6 ounces	1½ vegetable + 1 fat	80

BRAND-NAME EXCHANGES (*continued*)

Breads and Crackers	Serving Size	Exchanges per Serving	Calories per Serving*
Pepperidge Farm®			
goldfish crackers—cheddar cheese, parmesan cheese, lightly salted, pizza, sesame-garlic, or taco	45 to 50 crackers	1 bread + 1½ fat	140
goldfish thins—cheddar cheese, rye, or lightly salted	6 crackers	1 bread + 1 fat	105
croutons—cheddar cheese	½ cup	1½ bread + 1 fat	130
croutons—plain, seasoned, or onion-garlic	½ cup	1½ bread + 1 fat	140
Sara Lee®			
cinnamon rolls	1 roll	1 bread + 1 fat	105
croissant rolls	1 roll	1 bread + 1 fat	109
Parker House rolls	1 roll	1 bread + ½ fat	73
poppy seed rolls	1 roll	½ bread + ½ fat	55
Nabisco			
graham crackers	4	1½ bread + ½ fat	120
vanilla wafers	5	1 bread + ½ fat	93
Premium saltine crackers	7	1 bread + .4 fat	84

			Calories per Serving*
Premium crackers unsalted			
tops**	7	1 bread + .4 fat	84
Ritz crackers**	8	1 bread + 1.4 fat	133
Triscuits**	5	1 bread + .7 fat	100
Zwieback toast**	3	1 bread + .4 fat	90

Cereals	Serving Size	Exchanges per Serving	Calories per Serving*
Nabisco			
Cream of Wheat**	2 tbsp.	1 bread	80
Spoon size shredded wheat**	1/3 cup	1 bread	55
100% Bran cereal**	6 tbsp.	1 bread + 1/3 fat	53
Team flakes cereal**	2/3 cup	1 bread	73

Miscellaneous	Serving Size	Exchanges per Serving	Calories per Serving*
Contadina or Hunts			
canned pizza sauce	1 cup	1½ bread + 1 fat	220
canned tomato sauce	1 cup	1 bread	70
canned tomato paste	3/4 cup	2 bread	140
canned tomato sauce special**	1 cup	1 bread	80
Nabisco			
Snack Mate Pasteurized Cheese spreads All flavors**	4 tsp.	½ meat	60

BRAND-NAME EXCHANGES (continued)

Desserts	Serving Size	Exchanges per Serving	Calories per Serving*
General Foods			
fruit-flavored gelatin (prepared)	½ cup	1 bread	80
low-calorie pudding (prepared with skim milk)	½ cup	½ milk + ½ bread	70

* Calories listed for Betty Crocker, Kraft, Mrs. Paul's, Birds Eye, Minute, Stove Top, Lipton, and Nestle have been added to the Better Homes and Gardens lists by Diabetes Forecast.

** Added to the list by Forecast based on information supplied by the manufacturer. Copyright © 1978, 1979 Better Homes and Gardens. Reprinted with permission from Diabetes Forecast, March–April, 1980, p. 27–28.

HOW SWEET IT IS

Aspartame

A protein sweetener 180 times as sweet as sucrose. Not available for consumer use in the United States. Studies are being done on its safety. Technically, aspartame is caloric; however, it is so sweet that the amount used per serving of food is likely to supply almost no calories.

Carob Powder
Carob flour

Produced by grinding the pod of the carob tree. Tastes similar to chocolate. 75 percent is made up of sucrose, glucose, and fructose, which are all caloric.

Cyclamates*

Noncaloric sweeteners approximately 30 times as sweet as sucrose. Cyclamates were banned from use in the United States in 1970 because of questions about their possible cancer- and tumor-causing properties. They are still used in some foreign countries, and the risk associated with moderate use is considered by many to be very small.

Dextrin

Chains of glucose molecules. Their effect on blood glucose has not been well evaluated, but may be similar to glucose. Caloric.

Dulcitol

A sugar alcohol. Caloric.

Fructose
Fruit sugar
Levulose

One of the most common naturally occurring sugars, particularly found in fruit and honey. It is not associated with a rapid and high rise in blood sugar in well-controlled diabetes. The sweetness of refined fructose varies, but under certain conditions it can be almost twice as sweet as sucrose. Caloric.

HOW SWEET IT IS *(continued)*

Glucose
Corn sugar
Dextrose
Grape Sugar

A naturally occurring sugar that normally causes a fast and high rise in blood sugar. About half as sweet as table sugar. Carbohydrates (starches) break down to glucose during digestion, as do all sugars eventually. Glucose is the form of sugar that the body uses for energy and other purposes, and it builds up in the blood if diabetes is poorly controlled. *Dextrose* is the commercial name for glucose and will often be seen on food labels, including those of some sugar substitutes. Caloric.

Glucose Syrups
Corn syrup
Corn syrup solids
Sorghum syrup
Starch syrup
Sugar cane syrup

Liquid sweeteners produced by the breakdown (hydrolyzation) of starch. They contain a mixture of glucose, maltose, and longer chains of glucose molecules and can be produced from a variety of starches (hence, the varied names). *Corn syrup solids* are the crystallized form of corn syrup. Caloric.

High Fructose Corn Syrups

Produced from corn syrups. They contain differing amounts of fructose, ranging from 42–90 percent. The remaining part of the syrup is primarily glucose. The effect of the highly refined type (90 percent fructose) on blood glucose has not been well evaluated, but, theoretically, it should not cause high and fast rises of glucose in the blood of people whose diabetes is well controlled. The 90 percent type is the only one that might prove to be an acceptable sweetener for diabetics. Caloric.

Honey Comb honey Creamed honey	A natural syrup that varies in sugar and flavor depending on many factors. **It is** primarily glucose (about 35 percent), fructose (about 40 percent), and water, and, by weight, is about 75 percent as sweet as sucrose. Additional glucose is sometimes added to some honeys. Caloric.
Lactose	Milk sugar. It comprises about 4.5 percent of cow milk. About 30 percent as sweet as sucrose. Caloric.
Maltose	Two glucose units linked together. It is only 30–50 percent as sweet as sucrose, but it rapidly breaks down to glucose in the intestinal tract. Caloric.
Mannitol	A naturally occurring sugar alcohol that causes less of a rise in blood sugar than do sucrose or glucose. It is about half as sweet as sucrose and is slowly absorbed into the blood. In large amounts, it can cause diarrhea. Caloric.
Maple Syrup Maple sugar	Made from the sap of the maple and other trees. It is mostly sucrose with some invert sugar (see sucrose) and trace amounts of other compounds. The crystallized syrup is *maple sugar*. Caloric.
Milk Chocolate Bitter chocolate Bittersweet chocolate	Produced by the addition of milk, sugar, and cocoa butter to bitter chocolate. *Milk chocolate* is approximately 43 percent sugar and *bittersweet chocolate* is about 40 percent sugar. The sugar is caloric.
Molasses Blackstrap Golden syrup Refiners' syrup Treacle Unsulphured	The sugar drawn from sugar crystals as they are refined into pure sucrose. Different types are usually produced during sucrose refinement. All types, however, contain 50–75 percent sugar (sucrose and invert sugar) and should generally be avoided by diabetics. The sugars are caloric.

Saccharin	The currently used *noncaloric* sweetener in the United States. It is about 375 times as sweet as sucrose. The Food and Drug Administration is trying to ban it.
Sorbitol	A naturally occurring sugar alcohol found in many plants; commercially produced from glucose. It is about half as sweet as sucrose and more slowly absorbed than glucose. In individuals whose diabetes is well controlled, it causes only a small post-meal rise in blood glucose. In large amounts it may cause diarrhea. It is widely used in the manufacture of dietetic foods and chewing gums. Caloric.
Sucrose Beet sugar Brown sugar Cane sugar Confectioner's sugar Invert sugar Powdered sugar Raw sugar Saccharose Sugar Table sugar Turbinado	A naturally occurring sugar that is composed of equal parts of glucose and fructose linked together. It is produced from sugar cane or sugar beets. *Invert sugar* is made of sucrose that has been broken down to equal parts of glucose and fructose (with some sucrose left intact). *Brown sugars, raw sugar,* and *Turbinado* all contain some molasses.

Sweetened Condensed Whole Milk Sweetened condensed skim milk Sweetened condensed whey	Produced by reducing the water content of milk by about half and adding sugar. The finished product is about 44 percent sucrose, which is caloric. This means a 14 oz. can of condensed whole milk contains the equivalent of 8 Tbsp. of sugar and 2½ cups of milk.
Xylitol	A naturally occurring sugar alcohol produced from xylose (bark sugar). It is slowly absorbed and causes less of a rise in blood sugar than does sucrose or glucose. Depending on how it is used, it is as sweet or less sweet than sucrose. It is believed to be less cavity inducing than other sugars. Large amounts can cause diarrhea, and questions about its safety have held up its use in all but a few products. Caloric.

* The sweeteners in italics are generally felt to be appropriate sweeteners for the diabetic individual, provided they are used according to the recommendations of a physician or dietitian.

Courtesy of Phyllis Crapo, R.D. and Margaret A. Powers, R.D., *Diabetes Forecast*, March–April, 1981, p. 24. Copyright 1980 by the American Diabetes Association. Reprinted from *Diabetes Forecast* with permission.

═══ INJECTION SITES ═══

Arms, Legs-thigh-calf, Hips, Abdomen

Rotation:

Moving in a straight line give each injection about one inch apart. After finishing a line, move to the next arm, leg, or hip.

Then return to the beginning dropping down one inch. If this is not done, scar tissue may form, due to the repeated irritation from insulin being injected in the same place. These areas could get large and bumpy or sunken. The raised places are called hypertrophy or insulin pads. The sunken places are called areas of atrophy.

Remember:

1. **Warm the insulin** to body temperature before injection by holding the insulin-filled syringe in your hand for a minute.

2. Remember to use the **correct mixture** of insulins.

3. **Rotate the injections** an inch apart, (from arm to arm, thigh to thigh, etc.) using other areas such as the abdomen and under the "wing" bones (scapulae) when needed.

   Do not give any shots in areas that feel firm to the touch. These areas should be allowed to rest for six months or more until the area feels soft to the touch.

   An injection may be given in any area where there is skin over muscle. There should be enough fatty tissue in which to give the insulin into.

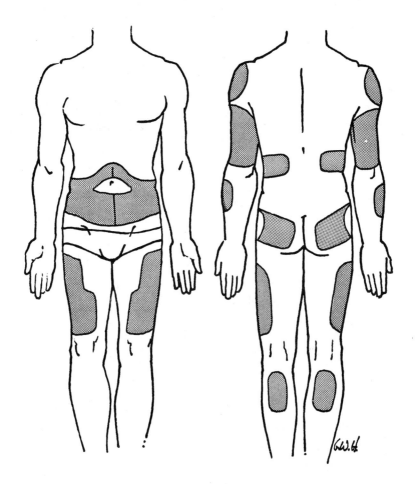

Injection sites are indicated in gray.

Courtesy of Diana Guthrie, Diabetes Nurse Specialist,
University of Kansas School of Medicine-Wichita

INSULIN ONSET, PEAK, AND ≡ EFFECTIVE DURATION ≡

INSULIN ONSET, PEAK, AND EFFECTIVE DURATION

Type of Insulin	Onset	Peak	Duration
Regular	Rapid (15–30 min.)	2–4	6–8
Semilente (amorphus)	Rapid (1 hour)	2–4+	6–8+
NPH	Intermediate 2–4	±2 hours 8	12–14
Lente (30% amorphus) (70% crystalline)	Intermediate 2–4	±2 hours 8	14–16
Globin	Intermediate 2–4	±2 hours 8	12–14
Protamine Zinc	Slow 4–6	18±	36–72
Ultralente (crystalline)	Very slow 8 hours	18±	24–36
Ilentin II (Pork) (Eli Lilly)	Same types as above		
Actrapid (Pork) (Novo)	Rapid	2½–5	6+
Velosulin (Quick) (Pork) (Nordisk)	Rapid	Like Regular	
Semitard (Pork) (Novo)	Rapid	Like Semilente	
Monotard (Pork) (Novo)	Intermediate	6–14	Like NPH

INSULIN ONSET, PEAK, AND EFFECTIVE DURATION
(continued)

Type of Insulin	Onset	Peak	Duration
Insulatard NPH (Pork) (Nordisk)	Intermediate	4–12	Like NPH
Lentard (Pork & Beef) (Novo)	Intermediate	6–14	Like Lente
Ultratard (Beef) (Novo)	Slow acting	10–30	Like Ultra Lente
Mixtard (Pork) (Nordisk)	Pre-Mixed Quick—33% NPH—67%		

Courtesy of Diana Guthrie, Diabetes Nurse Specialist, University of Kansas School of Medicine—Wichita

INSULINS SOLD IN THE U.S.

Insulin Type	Products (impurity level)*	Maker**	Brand Name
Rapid Acting†			
Regular	Purified Pork (<10 ppm)	Novo††	Actrapid
		Lilly	Iletin II, Pork
		Nordisk	Velosulin Quick
	Purified Beef (<10 ppm)	Lilly	Iletin II, Beef
	Beef-Pork (<50 ppm)	Lilly	Iletin I†††
	Beef-Pork (app. 10,000 ppm)	Squibb	Regular
Semilente	Purified Pork (<10 ppm)	Novo	Semitard
	Beef-Pork (<50 ppm)	Lilly	Iletin I
	Beef (app. 10,000 ppm)	Squibb	Semilente
30% Regular-70% Nph	Purified Pork (<10 ppm)	Nordisk	Mixtard
Intermediate Acting†			
Nph (Neutral Protamine Hagedorn)	Purified Pork (<10 ppm)	Lilly	Iletin II, Pork
		Nordisk	Insultard
	Purified Beef (<10 ppm)	Lilly	Iletin II, Beef
	Beef-Pork (<50 ppm)	Lilly	Iletin I
	Beef-Pork (app. 10,000 ppm)	Squibb	NPH
	Purified Pork (<10 ppm)	Lilly	Iletin II, Pork
Lente		Novo	Monotard
	Purified Beef (<10 ppm)	Lilly	Iletin II, Beef
	Purified Beef-Pork (<10 ppm)	Novo	Lentard
	Beef-Pork (<50 ppm)	Lilly	Iletin I

Globin	Beef-Pork (app. 10,000 ppm)	Squibb	Lente
	Beef-Pork (app. 10,000 ppm)	Squibb	Globin
Prolonged Acting†			
Pzi (Protamine-Zinc, Insulin)	Purified Pork ($<$10 ppm)	Lilly	Iletin II, Pork
	Purified Beef ($<$10 ppm)	Lilly	Iletin II, Beef
	Beef-Pork ($<$50 ppm)	Lilly	Iletin I
	Beef-Pork (app. 10,000 ppm)	Squibb	PZI
Ultralente	Purified Beef ($<$10 ppm)	Novo	Ultratard
	Beef-Pork ($<$50 ppm)	Lilly	Iletin I
	Beef (app. 10,000 ppm)	Squibb	Ultralente

*Measured by parts of proinsulin per million parts of insulin (ppm); $<$ means "less than."

**All Novo and Nordisk insulins are sold in U-100 concentration only. Lilly's Iletin®I insulins are available in U-100 and U-40. Squibb's products are all available in U-100; Regular, Lente, and NPH are also sold in U-40.

†The speed and duration of insulin action may vary from product to product.

††FDA standards for using the term "highly purified" is impurities of fewer than 10 ppm. Novo's products actually contain impurities of 1 ppm or less, but no one knows whether variations in purity within the "highly purified" category have any effect on health.

†††Formerly called Improved Single Peak Iletin.

Copyright 1981 by the American Diabetes Association. Reprinted from *Diabetes Forecast* with permission.

235

GLUCAGON FOR EMERGENCY TREATMENT OF INSULIN SHOCK

Description. Glucagon is a protein hormone produced normally in the body by specialized cells of the pancreas called the alpha cells of the islands of Langerhans. Glucagon and insulin have opposite effects; insulin lowers blood sugar, whereas glucagon raises blood sugar.

The drug is prepared commercially from animal pancreas and is available, by prescription only, in a two-bottle kit. One bottle contains the purified glucagon in dry powder form, and the other contains a diluting solution.

Action. Glucagon causes an increase in blood glucose concentration and, therefore, is used in the treatment of hypoglycemic states (low blood sugar) called insulin reaction or insulin shock. Glucagon acts by changing stored sugar in the liver (glycogen) to a usable form of sugar (glucose).

Indications. Glucagon is useful in counteracting severe hypoglycemic reactions *due to insulin* in diabetics who are unable to take food or drink by mouth. The sooner after the onset of a reaction that glucagon is administered, the greater the likelihood of its being effective.

Adverse Reactions. Glucagon is relatively free of undesirable side effects, except for occasional upset stomach, nausea, and vomiting. There is no danger of overdosage with glucagon; it is a safe drug.

Courtesy of the American Diabetes Association, Inc.

For the user's information: General directions for use

Glucagon is an emergency drug to be used only under the direction of a physician. Become familiar with the following instructions before the emergency arises.

In case of insulin coma or severe reactions, administer glucagon and call a physician promptly.

Act quickly. Unconsciousness over a period of time may be very harmful.

Inject glucagon in the same way that insulin is injected (see following directions). Turn patient to one side or face down. Rest face on arms.

The patient usually awakens within 15 minutes. Feed the patient as soon as he awakens.

Glucagon is a safe drug. There is no danger of overdosage.

Note: Glucagon should not be prepared for injection until the emergency arises.

To prepare glucagon for injection

1. Remove the flip-off seals on bottles Nos. 1 and 2.

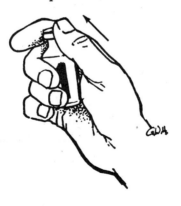

2. Wipe the rubber stoppers on both bottles with a suitable antiseptic if available (alcohol or isopropyl alcohol).

3. Use a U-40 or U-100 insulin syringe and needle.

4. Draw the plunger of the syringe back to the 20-unit mark on a U-40 syringe or to the 50-unit mark on a U-100 syringe.

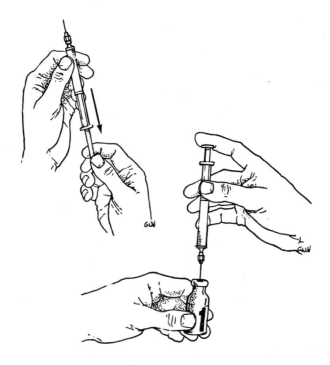

5. Pick up the smaller, white-labeled bottle (No. 1) containing the diluting solution. Pierce the center of the stopper with the needle attached to the syringe.

6. Turn the bottle upside down and inject the air from the syringe into the bottle. It will then be possible to remove the diluting solution more easily.

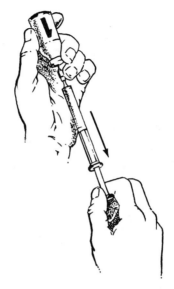

7. Keep the tip of the needle in the diluting solution and withdraw as much of the solution as possible into the syringe.

8. Remove the needle and syringe from bottle No. 1 and insert this same needle into the bottle (No. 2) containing the glucagon. Inject all of the diluting solution from the syringe into bottle No. 2.

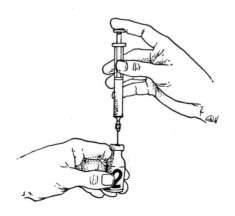

9. Remove needle and syringe. Shake bottle gently. The glucagon will dissolve, and the preparation will become clear. Withdraw the entire contents of the bottle into the syringe. The solution is now ready for injection into the patient.

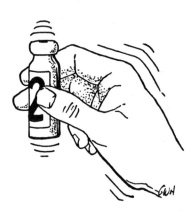

To administer glucagon use same technique as for injecting insulin

The remaining steps are the same as those for injecting insulin

10. Select the injection site. Glucagon is administered like insulin. It can be given in the abdomen, buttocks, upper and outer thigh, or the back, fatty part of the upper arm.

11. Wipe the site with cotton dipped in alcohol.

12. Pinch up the area of skin and fat to be injected.

13. Inject needle through skin. (A 90° angle is satisfactory unless the diabetic is extremely thin. In that case, use a 45° angle.)

14. Push on plunger to inject the entire amount of glucagon. (If the person being treated is under three years old, use only one-half the dose.)

15. Withdraw the needle from the skin.

16. Press the cotton gently on the injection site.

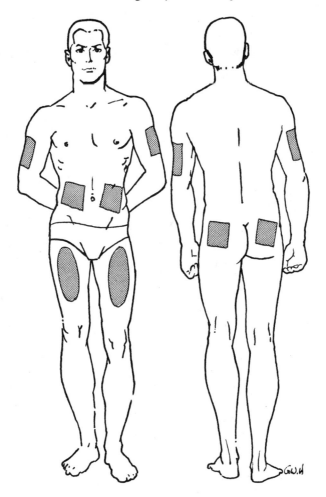

Injection sites are indicated in gray.

When treated with glucagon, the severe hypoglycemic state usually subsides, and the diabetic awakens within 15 minutes. If the unconscious diabetic vomits as he is waking up, he should be turned face down on one side to help prevent breathing any stomach contents into his lungs.

As soon as the patient is alert enough to swallow, feed him some carbohydrate! (Examples of quick carbohydrate sources include soft drinks, orange juice, and sugar dissolved in water.) This should be followed by a longer-acting carbohydrate, such as a cracker or a sandwich, to avoid a second hypoglycemic episode, since glucagon acts for only a short period of time.

Other Instructions. If the unconscious diabetic does not awaken within 20 minutes, the dose may be repeated, and a physician should be consulted as soon as possible.

If you find the diabetic unconscious and are not sure whether his comatose condition is due to high (hyper-) or low (hypo-) blood sugar, it is best to assume this is a low (hypo-) blood sugar state and to give glucagon.

Do not use the glucagon after the date stamped on the label of bottle No. 2.

How Supplied. Glucagon is available in two package sizes: a single-dose kit containing 1 unit (1 mg) of glucagon, intended for use by the diabetic; a 10-unit (10-mg) multidose package, intended for institutional use.

Where Available. Glucagon is a prescription drug available at most pharmacies. The cost varies from one drugstore to another. Ask your doctor to prescribe it for you.

INSULIN REACTION
INFORMATION

(Slow onset)
high blood sugar
diabetic acidosis
hyperglycemia

Watch for:

Increased thirst and urination

Large amounts of sugar and ketones in urine

Weakness, abdominal pains, generalized aches

Loss of appetite, nausea, and vomiting

Heavy labored breathing

What to do:

Call doctor

Give patient fluids without sugar if able to swallow

Continue usual urine tests

Causes:

Too little insulin

Failure to follow diet

Infection, fever

Emotional stress

(Rapid onset) low blood sugar insulin reaction hypoglycemia

Watch for:

Excessive sweating, faintness

Headache

Pounding of heart, trembling, impaired vision

Hunger

Not able to awaken

Irritability

Personality change

What to do:

Give sugar, or food containing sugar (honey, candy, fruit)

Do not give fluid if patient is not conscious

Do not give insulin

Give glucagon if loss of consciousness

Call doctor

Causes:

Too much insulin

Not eating enough food

Unusual amount of exercise

Delayed meal

Produced by Becton Dickinson Consumer Products, Rochelle Park, New Jersey 07622.

SUGGESTED READING

BOOKS

Anderson, James W.; Sieling, Beverly; and Chen, Wen-Ju Lin. *User's Guide to HCF Diets.* Lexington: HCF Diabetes Research Fund, Inc., 1980.

A high-carbohydrate, high-fiber, low-fat diet plan developed at the University of Kentucky. Reduces insulin requirements and provides other major health benefits for all diabetics.

Bernstein, Richard K. *Diabetes: The Glucograf Method for Normalizing Blood Sugar.* New York: Crown, 1981.

Bernstein, an insulin-dependent diabetic for 35 years, originated the Glucograf method, which keeps blood sugar normal 90 percent of the time and which, according to his theory, will eliminate the long-range complications of diabetes. This book is a step-by-step guide to his admittedly rigorous regime. (Sponsored by the Diabetes Research and Training Center of the Albert Einstein College of Medicine and Montefiore Hospital and Medical Center in New York.)

Biermann, June, and Toohey, Barbara. *The Diabetic's Sports and Exercise Book.* Philadelphia and New York: Lippincott, 1977.

How to play your way to better health. Over 150 diabetics share their sports experiences from lawn bowling to scuba diving. The secrets of using exercise to improve your diabetes control *and* your life.

Biermann, June, and Toohey, Barbara. *The Diabetic's Total Health Book.* Los Angeles: J. P. Tarcher, 1980.

Learning to concentrate on your health rather than on your disease. Includes latest breakthroughs in day-to-day diabetes care: home blood sugar testing; high-carbohydrate, high-fiber diet; stress reduction; lifestyle changing. Working in partnership with your doctor for a strong body, a tranquil mind and a blithe spirit.

Biermann, June, and Toohey, Barbara. *The Peripatetic Diabetic.* New York: Hawthorn Books, 1969.

Overcoming the despair of diabetes and learning to live a joyful and exciting life; dining (lots of international gourmet recipes), travel, and general good times.

Directory of Medical Specialists, 1977-78. 18th edition. Chicago: Marquis Who's Who, Inc., 1979.

Lists the specialists in all fields of medicine by state and city and tells their education and experience.

Dosti, Rose: Kidushim, Deborah; and Wolke, Mark. *Light Style: The New American Cuisine.* San Francisco: Harper & Row, 1979.

Over 250 delicious low-calorie recipes, each followed by a listing of calorie, cholesterol, salt and fat content plus diabetic exchanges. Sweeteners are mainly fructose or fruit.

Graedon, Joe. *The People's Pharmacy.* New York: Avon, 1976. *The People's Pharmacy—Two.* New York: Avon, 1980.

Indispensable guides to prescription drugs, dangerous drug interactions, brand-name medications, and money-saving home remedies.

Jacobson, Michel F. *Eater's Digest; The Consumer's Factbook of Food Additives.* Garden City, N.Y.: Doubleday & Co., Inc., 1972.

The book to put you on guard against all the nasties that are thrown into processed food.

Jones, Jeanne. *The Calculating Cook.* San Francisco: 101 Productions, 1972. *More Calculated Cooking.* San Francisco: 101 Productions, 1981.

Jeanne Jones, herself a diabetic and gourmet cook, has combined her experience and talents to produce these two excellent cookbooks that not only help you stay on your diet but make dining a joy. No strange tasting diabetic gunk or hospital fare here!

Krall, Leo J., editor. *Joslin Diabetes Manual.* 11th edition. Philadelphia: Lea & Febiger, 1978.

The manual from Boston's famed Joslin Clinic. This is a kind of postgraduate course for diabetics who want to know the scientific whys behind the hows of diabetes care.

Majors, Judith S. *Sugarfree Kids' Cookery.* Milwaukie, Oregon: Apple Press, 1979.

A collection of calculated recipes with child appeal, simple enough for a young diabetic to prepare. Many dishes are state and county fair ribbon winners. (Approved by the ADA Oregon Affiliate.)

Majors, Judith S. *Sugar Free . . . Microwavery Calculated Cookbook.* Milwaukie, Oregon: Apple Press, 1980.

Microwave cooking is quick and easy and eliminates fat in foods. The author, a diabetic who claims she lives to eat, has converted 140 favorite recipes to microwave and has calculated exchanges for each. (Approved by the ADA Oregon Affiliate.)

Peterson, Charles M. *Take Charge of Your Diabetes: A New Approach to Self-Management.* Author, 1979. (Available from Take Charge of Your Diabetes, Just Mailings, P.O. Box 802, South Bend, Indiana 46624, $3.95.)

A short but complete manual on how to keep good control of your diabetes by using reagent sticks and a meter to take your own blood sugar.

Robertson, Laurel; Flinders, Carol; and Godfrey, Bronwen. *Laurel's Kitchen.* New York: Bantam Books, 1976.

For the diabetic who wants to be a vegetarian or simply wants to eat a more healthful diet. Beautiful philosophy, delicious recipes, and the most accurate and understandable of scientific information. This is as nearly perfect as a cookbook can be.

Sims, Dorothea, editor. *Diabetes: Reach for Health and Freedom.* St. Louis: C. V. Mosby, 1980. (Available from C. V. Mosby Company, 11830 Westline Industrial Drive, St. Louis, MO 63141, $5.95.)

A lucid, upbeat manual of self-care, emphasizing options rather than rules. Written by a team of health professionals and an editor who has had diabetes for over 25 years.

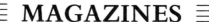

MAGAZINES

Diabetes Care
2 Park Avenue
New York, NY 10016

Bimonthly magazine for doctors and other members of the health-care team specializing in diabetes.

Aimed at improving the care of patients with diabetes. Published by the American Diabetes Association. Subscription rate is $25.00 per year.

Diabetes Forecast
2 Park Avenue
New York, NY 10016

Bimonthly magazine for diabetics published by the American Diabetes Association. Subscription rate $6.00 per year or included in membership in the American Diabetes Association.

Diabetes in the News
233 East Erie Street, Suite 712
Chicago, IL 60611

Bimonthly newspaper for diabetics. Write for free subscription.

INDEX

INDEX